CHRISTY LYNN

Top 50+ exercises for Senior Adults

Gain muscle, increase balance, look & feel better in your own skin.

Contents

1

Chapter 1

Understanding Senior Fitness

As we journey through life, our bodies undergo a natural transformation, and with each passing year, maintaining our health becomes increasingly vital. For seniors, the significance of fitness extends far beyond aesthetics; it becomes a cornerstone for overall well-being. In this chapter, we delve into the fundamental reasons why fitness holds such paramount importance in the lives of seniors, exploring the physical, mental, and emotional facets of exercise tailored to this demographic.

Physical Benefits of Exercise for Seniors

Age doesn't define our potential for physical prowess. Seniors engaging in regular physical activity experience a remarkable array of benefits. From enhanced cardiovascular health and improved flexibility to the preservation of muscle mass and bone density, exercise is the key to counteracting the natural decline that comes with aging. Studies by esteemed institutions consistently affirm that even moderate exercise significantly reduces the risk of chronic illnesses like heart disease, diabetes, and osteoporosis among seniors.

Mental and Emotional Well-being

Beyond the physical realm, exercise profoundly impacts mental and emotional health. Seniors who engage in routine exercise report heightened cognitive function, better memory retention, and a reduced risk of cognitive decline. Moreover, the release of endorphins through physical activity elevates mood, mitigating stress, anxiety, and depression. It fosters a sense of accomplishment, boosting self-esteem and confidence, vital elements in leading a fulfilling life in the golden years.

Common Concerns and Misconceptions

Yet, amidst the vast array of benefits, common concerns and misconceptions often deter seniors from embracing exercise. Addressing these apprehensions is crucial. Debunking myths such as "it's too late to start" or "exercise might cause injury" is imperative. By carefully highlighting the adaptability and safety of tailored fitness routines, seniors can approach exercise with confidence and a clearer understanding of their capabilities.

Physical Benefits of Exercise for Seniors

• **Heart Health:** Regular exercise helps keep the heart strong and healthy. It makes the heart muscles stronger, allowing it to pump blood more efficiently. This lowers the risk of heart diseases like heart attacks and strokes.

• **Improved Flexibility:** Doing exercises like stretching or yoga helps seniors stay flexible. It keeps the body limber and makes it easier to move around, reducing the chances of muscle strains or falls.

• **Stronger Bones and Muscles:** When seniors exercise, it helps keep their bones and muscles strong. This is super important because it reduces the risk of fractures and helps them stay independent and active.

• **Better Balance and Coordination**: Exercise, especially activities that focus on balance, like tai chi or specific strengthening exercises, helps seniors improve their balance. This means fewer falls and accidents, keeping them safe.

• **Reduced Joint Pain**: Contrary to what some might think, gentle exercise can actually ease joint pain for seniors. Activities like swimming or biking are easy on the joints, relieving pain and stiffness while keeping them active.

• **Increased Energy Levels:** Regular physical activity boosts energy levels in seniors. It might seem paradoxical, but the more they move, the more energy they have, allowing them to do more activities throughout the day without feeling tired.

These benefits show how exercise isn't just about muscles and sweat; it's about keeping the body strong, flexible, and able to handle day-to-day activities without discomfort or the risk of injuries.

Mental and Emotional Well-being from Exercise

• **Sharper Mind**: Exercise keeps the brain in good shape. It helps seniors stay focused, remember things better, and can even slow down memory loss.

• **Mood Booster:** When seniors exercise, their brains release happy chemicals called endorphins. This can make them feel happier, less stressed, and more relaxed.

• **Confidence Booster:** Seeing progress in their fitness can boost confidence. Seniors feel proud of what they achieve, which can improve self-esteem and make them feel more capable.

• **Stress Buster:** Exercise is like a stress-relief button. It helps seniors cope better with stress and can reduce feelings of anxiety or sadness.

• **Social Connections:** Some exercises, like group classes or walking clubs, help seniors connect with others. Socializing while exercising can lift their spirits and reduce feelings of loneliness.

• **Better Sleep:** Regular exercise can improve sleep quality. Seniors might find it easier to fall asleep and stay asleep, waking up feeling more refreshed.

Exercise isn't just about the body; it's a powerful tool for keeping the mind happy and healthy. It's like giving the brain a workout that pays off in feelings of happiness and mental sharpness.

Common Concerns and Misconceptions about Exercise for Seniors

• **"It's Too Late to Start Exercising":** Some seniors worry that since they haven't exercised much before, it's too late to start. But starting exercise at any age can bring benefits. It's never too late to improve strength, flexibility, and overall health. Starting exercise later in life can still improve health, strengthen muscles, and boost energy levels.

• **"Exercise Might Cause Injury":** There's a fear that exercise could lead to injuries, especially in older bodies. However, starting with gentle exercises and gradually increasing intensity can greatly reduce the risk of injury. Gentle exercises tailored to abilities can improve health without causing harm.

• **"I Have Health Issues, Exercise Is Risky"**: Some seniors with health issues worry that exercise might make things worse. However, with guidance from healthcare professionals, many can find suitable exercises that won't aggravate existing conditions. Properly chosen exercises, considering health conditions, can actually improve overall well-being.

• **"I'm Not Fit Enough to Exercise"**: Seniors might feel they're not fit enough for exercise. Yet, there are plenty of exercises suited for various fitness levels, offering gradual progression. Starting with exercises that match current fitness levels can build strength and confidence gradually.

• **"Exercise Requires Expensive Equipment or Gym Memberships"**: Some believe exercise demands costly equipment or gym memberships. However, simple, effective exercises often require minimal or no equipment, making it accessible for everyone. Cost-effective exercises can be performed at home, outdoors, or in community centers, making fitness accessible to all.

Addressing these concerns and misconceptions can help us understand that exercise isn't a risky or daunting task. Instead, it's an adaptable and beneficial tool for improving health and well-being, regardless of age or fitness level.

2

Chapter 2

Safety

Understanding how to exercise safely is crucial, especially for seniors. This chapter will focus on why safety matters and provide essential guidelines for exercising without risking injury.

Pre-Exercise Health Check

Before diving into exercise, it's crucial to perform a health check. This involves assessing current health conditions, existing injuries, or any recent surgeries. Checking with a healthcare provider or a fitness professional is recommended to ensure exercise choices align with individual health conditions and limitations.

Proper Warm-Up and Cool-Down Techniques

Proper warm-up and cool-down routines are key to a safe and effective exercise regimen. Explaining the significance of these routines and providing simple, senior-friendly warm-up and cool-down exercises will help prevent strains and enhance flexibility.

Considerations for Seniors with Health Conditions

Seniors often have specific health concerns that need special attention during exercise. Addressing these considerations, such as arthritis, osteoporosis, diabetes, or heart conditions, will guide them on exercising safely. It's important to emphasize modifications or exercises tailored to accommodate these conditions without exacerbating them.

This chapter aims to equip seniors with the knowledge and tools necessary to exercise safely. By understanding the importance of safety measures and incorporating them into their workout routines, they can enjoy the benefits of exercise without risking their well-being.

Pre-Exercise Health Check

• **Medical History Review:** Look at your medical history, including any previous surgeries, injuries, or chronic health conditions. Knowing this helps plan exercises that suit your body's needs and limitations. Understanding your medical history helps avoid exercises that might cause harm or discomfort due to previous injuries or conditions.

• **Consultation with a Healthcare Provider:** Talk to your doctor or a fitness professional before starting any new exercise routine, especially if you have health concerns. They can offer personalized advice and ensure your chosen exercises align with your health needs. Getting professional advice ensures exercise choices are safe and suitable for your specific health conditions.

• **Assessment of Current Physical Condition**: Consider your current physical state, including strength, flexibility, and stamina. This self-assessment helps in selecting exercises that match your fitness level, avoiding overexertion or injuries. Choosing exercises that match your current fitness level helps prevent strain or injury during workouts.

• **Awareness of Pain or Discomfort:** Be aware of any pain, discomfort, or unusual sensations during daily activities. This awareness helps identify areas that need caution or specific exercises to avoid aggravating discomfort. Recognizing pain or discomfort allows adjustments to exercise routines to prevent worsening conditions.

• **Understanding Exercise Goals and Limitations**: Clearly define what you want to achieve with your exercises and acknowledge any physical limitations or restrictions. Setting realistic goals helps tailor exercises that align with your capabilities. Having clear exercise goals and knowing your limits helps create an exercise routine that's safe, effective, and enjoyable.

By conducting a thorough pre-exercise health check, individuals can better understand their bodies, health constraints, and capabilities. This knowledge forms the foundation for designing a safe and personalized exercise regimen.

Proper Warm-Up and Cool-Down Techniques

• **Dynamic Stretching**: Start with dynamic stretches like arm circles, leg swings, or torso twists. These movements help increase blood flow and loosen up muscles, preparing them for more intense exercises. Benefit: Dynamic stretches help prevent injury by gradually preparing muscles and joints for movement.

• **Light Cardio Exercises:** Begin with five to ten minutes of low-intensity cardio, like brisk walking or cycling. This elevates the heart rate and warms up the body, priming it for more vigorous activity. Benefit: Light cardio raises body temperature and oxygenates muscles, reducing the risk of strain during exercise.

• **Joint Mobilization Exercises:** Perform gentle movements that focus on the joints, such as ankle rolls, shoulder rotations, or wrist bends. This enhances joint flexibility and lubrication, reducing the risk of stiffness or injury. Benefit: Mobilizing joints before exercise helps improve flexibility and range of motion, preventing joint discomfort.

• **Foam Rolling or Self-Massage:** Use a foam roller or perform self-massage on tight areas or muscles prone to tension. This helps release knots and tension, improving muscle elasticity and readiness for exercise. Benefit: Foam rolling, or self-massage relaxes muscles and increases blood flow, reducing the likelihood of muscle strain.

• **Gradual Cooling Down**: After exercise, gradually reduce the intensity of the workout for around 5-10 minutes. This could include walking or stretching. Cooling down slowly helps the heart rate return to normal gradually. Benefit: Gradual cooling down prevents dizziness and lightheadedness by allowing the body to adjust from exercise intensity to a resting state.

Proper warm-up and cool-down techniques are essential components of an exercise routine. They prepare the body for physical activity, reduce the risk of injury, and aid in a smooth transition from exercise to rest, optimizing overall workout effectiveness.

Considerations for Seniors with Health Conditions

• Arthritis: For seniors dealing with arthritis, low-impact exercises like swimming or cycling can reduce joint stress while improving mobility and strength. Benefit: Low-impact exercises help maintain joint health without worsening arthritis symptoms.

• Osteoporosis: Weight-bearing exercises, such as walking or dancing, strengthen bones for seniors with osteoporosis, reducing the risk of fractures. Benefit: Weight-bearing exercises can enhance bone density, decreasing the chances of fractures.

• Diabetes: Seniors with diabetes benefit from aerobic exercises like brisk walking or cycling, as these activities help control blood sugar levels and improve heart health. Benefit: Aerobic exercises contribute to better blood sugar management and cardiovascular health for those with diabetes.

• Heart Conditions: Light cardio exercises and supervised routines tailored to individual heart conditions help improve cardiovascular health without straining the heart excessively. Benefit: Customized exercise plans support heart health without putting excess stress on the heart.

• Balance Issues: Seniors experiencing balance problems can benefit from exercises like Tai Chi or yoga, as these activities enhance balance and stability. Benefit: Balance-focused exercises improve stability, reducing the risk of falls and related injuries.

Understanding how different health conditions interact with exercise is crucial for seniors. Tailoring exercise routines to accommodate these conditions helps improve overall health while minimizing the risk of exacerbating specific health issues.

3

Chapter 3

Warm-up and Mobility Exercises

Neck and Shoulder Mobility

• **Neck Rotations:** Slowly turn your head to the right, then to the left, keeping movements gentle. This exercise increases neck flexibility, reducing stiffness and enhancing range of motion. Benefit: Alleviates tension and stiffness, improving neck flexibility and reducing discomfort.

• **Shoulder Rolls:** Lift shoulders towards ears, roll them back and down in circular motions. This motion loosens shoulder muscles, easing tightness and enhancing shoulder joint mobility. Benefit: Releases shoulder tension, improving flexibility and reducing discomfort.

• **Neck Tilts**: Gently tilt your head to the right, then to the left, feeling the stretch along the sides of your neck. This exercise stretches neck muscles, enhancing flexibility and reducing strain. Benefit: Relieves neck tension and enhances flexibility, reducing stiffness.

• **Shoulder Blade Squeezes:** Sit or stand tall, gently squeeze shoulder blades together. This action strengthens upper back muscles, promoting better posture. Benefit: Strengthens upper back, aiding posture and reducing slouching.

• **Shoulder Stretch Across Body**: Bring right arm across the body, gently press right elbow with left hand, feeling a stretch in the shoulder. Repeat on the other side. This stretch improves shoulder flexibility and reduces tension. Benefit: Enhances shoulder flexibility, reduces tightness, and improves range of motion.

• **Neck Flexion and Extension:** Slowly bring your chin towards your chest, then look up towards the ceiling, keeping movements gentle. This exercise stretches the front and back of the neck, improving flexibility. Benefit: Enhances neck flexibility, reduces stiffness, and increases mobility.

• **Shoulder Circles**: Rotate shoulders forward in circular motions, then backward. This exercise improves shoulder joint mobility and reduces stiffness. Benefit: Enhances shoulder mobility, loosens muscles, and reduces discomfort.

• **Upper Trapezius Stretch**: Gently tilt your head towards one shoulder, feeling a stretch along the side of the neck and shoulder. Repeat on the other side. This stretch reduces tension in the upper trapezius muscles. Benefit: Relieves tension in the upper trapezius muscles, reducing tightness and discomfort.

**These exercises aim to increase flexibility, reduce stiffness, and enhance mobility in the neck and shoulders, contributing to improved comfort and reduced risk of strain or injury in these areas.

Ankles

• **Ankle Circles:** Lift one foot and rotate your ankle clockwise, then counterclockwise. This exercise increases ankle flexibility, reduces stiffness, and enhances range of motion. Benefit: Improves ankle flexibility, reducing stiffness, and making movements smoother.

• **Toe Flexion and Extension:** Sit on a chair, raise one foot, then point your toes forward and then pull them back towards your shin. This exercise strengthens ankle muscles and improves flexibility. Benefit: Strengthens ankle muscles and increases flexibility, reducing the risk of injuries.

• **Calf Raises:** Stand with feet shoulder-width apart, rise up on your toes, then slowly lower back down. This exercise strengthens calf muscles, improving ankle stability. Benefit: Strengthens calf muscles, enhancing ankle support and stability.

• **Alphabet Writing with Toes:** While sitting or lying down, lift one foot and write the alphabet in the air with your toes. This exercise improves ankle mobility and flexibility. Benefit: Enhances ankle mobility and flexibility, promoting better range of motion.

• **Resistance Band Ankle Flexion and Extension:** Sit on the floor with a resistance band looped around the ball of one foot, then flex and point your foot against the band's resistance. This exercise strengthens ankle muscles. Benefit: Strengthens ankle muscles, improving stability and reducing the risk of twists or sprains.

• **Towel Scrunches:** Place a towel on the floor, and using your toes, scrunch the towel towards you. This exercise strengthens toe and ankle muscles, improving control and stability. Benefit: Strengthens toe and ankle muscles, enhancing control and stability.

• **Heel Raises:** Stand with feet flat on the floor, then raise your heels off the ground, lifting onto the balls of your feet. This exercise strengthens ankle muscles, improving balance. Benefit: Strengthens ankle muscles, enhancing balance and stability.

• **Ankle Dorsiflexion Stretch:** Sit on the floor, loop a resistance band around your foot, gently pulling your toes towards you to feel a stretch in your calf and ankle. This stretch increases ankle flexibility. Benefit: Enhances ankle flexibility, reducing tightness and discomfort in the calf and ankle.

**These exercises aim to improve ankle strength, flexibility, and mobility, reducing the risk of injuries and enhancing overall stability during movements.

Hips

• **Hip Circles:** Stand with hands on hips, slowly rotate hips clockwise and then counterclockwise. This exercise increases hip mobility, reduces stiffness, and improves range of motion. Benefit: Enhances hip flexibility, reducing stiffness and improving movement.

• **Leg Swings:** Hold onto a sturdy surface and swing one leg forward and backward. This exercise loosens hip muscles, improves flexibility, and enhances hip joint mobility. Benefit: Loosens hip muscles, making them more flexible and mobile.

• **Hip Flexor Stretch:** Kneel on one knee, lunge forward, feeling a stretch in the front of your hip. Alternate legs. **This stretch increases hip flexibility and eases tightness in the hip flexors. Benefit: Increases hip flexibility, reduces tightness, and discomfort in the front of the hip.

• **Butterfly Stretch:** Sit on the floor, bring feet together, and gently press knees toward the ground. This stretch opens up the hips and improves flexibility in the inner thighs. Benefit: Opens hips, improves inner thigh flexibility, and reduces stiffness.

• **Lateral Leg Raises**: Lie on your side, lift the top leg up, then lower it back down. This exercise strengthens hip muscles, enhancing stability and reducing the risk of hip-related issues. Benefit: Strengthens hip muscles, improving stability and reducing the chance of hip problems.

• **Hip Rotations in Sitting:** Sit on a chair, cross one ankle over the opposite knee, then gently push the crossed knee down towards the floor. This exercise increases hip rotation and flexibility. Benefit: Enhances hip rotation and flexibility, improving overall hip mobility.

• **Hip Abduction:** Lie on your side, then lift the top leg up and slowly lower it back down. This exercise strengthens outer hip muscles, aiding stability and reducing strain. Benefit: Strengthens outer hip muscles, enhancing stability and reducing stress on the hips.

• **Hip Extension:** Stand tall, then slowly lift one leg backward, keeping the knee straight. This exercise strengthens hip muscles and improves balance. Benefit: Strengthens hip muscles, improving balance and reducing the risk of hip issues.

**These exercises focus on improving hip flexibility, strength, and mobility, which helps reduce stiffness, improve range of motion, and lower the risk of hip-related discomfort or injuries.

Gentle Dynamic Stretches

• **Arm Circles:** Extend your arms out to the sides and make small circles forward, then backward. This stretch warms up the shoulder muscles, improving flexibility and reducing tension. Benefit: Warms up shoulder muscles, making them more flexible and easing tension.

• **Torso Twists:** Stand with feet shoulder-width apart, gently twist your torso from side to side. This stretch helps loosen the spine and improve torso flexibility. Benefit: Loosens the spine and improves flexibility in the torso.

• **Leg Swings (Forward and Backward):** Hold onto a stable surface and swing one leg forward and backward. This movement helps to increase hip mobility and loosens leg muscles. Benefit: Increases hip mobility and loosens leg muscles for improved flexibility.

• **Side Bends:** Stand with feet hip-width apart and gently lean sideways, reaching one arm overhead. This stretch works on the side muscles of the body, improving flexibility. Benefit: Stretches side muscles, improving overall flexibility.

• **Ankle Bounces:** Stand tall and lightly bounce up and down on the balls of your feet. This exercise loosens up calf muscles and improves ankle flexibility.

• Benefit: Loosens calf muscles and increases ankle flexibility.

• **Shoulder Rolls with Reach:** Roll your shoulders back and down while reaching your arms up overhead. This movement stretches the shoulder muscles and upper back. Benefit: Stretches shoulder muscles and upper back, enhancing flexibility.

• **Hip Circles:** Stand with feet apart and make circular motions with your hips, clockwise and counterclockwise. This stretch improves hip mobility and reduces stiffness.Benefit: Improves hip mobility and reduces hip stiffness.

• **Neck Tilts and Rotations:** Gently tilt your head to the sides and rotate it in circular motions. This exercise reduces tension in the neck and improves neck flexibility.Benefit: Reduces tension in the neck and enhances neck flexibility.

• **Marching in Place:** Lift your knees high as if marching while standing in place. This movement helps to warm up the leg muscles and improve circulation. Benefit: Warms up leg muscles and enhances circulation.

•

• **Full Body Swings:** Stand with feet wide apart and swing arms from side to side, letting your torso follow the movement. This stretch works on overall body flexibility.

• Benefit: Works on overall body flexibility, stretching multiple muscles.

**These gentle dynamic stretches aim to warm up muscles, improve flexibility, and reduce tension in various parts of the body, helping to prepare for more intensive physical activities while reducing the risk of injury.

More Gentle Dynamic Stretches

• **Arm Swings:** Swing your arms forward and backward alternately, gently increasing the range of motion. This stretch warms up shoulder joints and improves flexibility in the upper body. Benefit: Warms up shoulder joints, enhances upper body flexibility.

• **Standing Side Leg Lifts:** While standing, lift one leg out to the side and then lower it back down. This movement improves hip flexibility and strengthens outer thigh muscles. Benefit: Improves hip flexibility, strengthens outer thigh muscles.

• **Wrist Circles:** Extend arms forward and rotate your wrists in circular motions, both clockwise and counterclockwise. This exercise loosens wrist joints and improves mobility in the wrists and forearms. Benefit: Loosens wrist joints, improves wrist and forearm mobility.

• **Seated Leg Extensions:** Sit on a chair, extend one leg forward, and flex and point your foot. This stretch targets the calf and hamstring muscles, improving leg flexibility. Benefit: Targets calf and hamstring muscles, enhances leg flexibility.

• **Dynamic Chest Stretch:** Stand tall, interlace fingers behind your back, and gently lift arms upward. This movement stretches the chest muscles and shoulders. Benefit: Stretches chest muscles and improves shoulder flexibility.

• **Knee Hugs:** Stand upright, bring one knee toward your chest, and hug it with both arms. This exercise helps in stretching the lower back and glutes. Benefit: Stretches lower back and glute muscles.

• **Heel-to-Toe Rocks:** Stand with feet together, gently rock backward onto your heels, then forward onto your toes. This stretch improves ankle flexibility and balance. Benefit: Enhances ankle flexibility and improves balance.

• **Ankle Alphabet:** Lift one foot and write the alphabet in the air using your big toe. This dynamic movement loosens up ankle joints and improves mobility. Benefit: Loosens ankle joints, enhances ankle mobility.

• **Pelvic Tilts:** Stand or sit, gently tilt your pelvis forward and backward. This movement helps to stretch and loosen lower back muscles. Benefit: Stretches and loosens lower back muscles.

• **Calf Stretch Walk:** Take small steps forward while pushing one heel to the ground at a time. This exercise stretches the calves and improves ankle flexibility. Benefit: Stretches calves and enhances ankle flexibility.

**These additional dynamic stretches aim to warm up different muscle groups, improve joint mobility, and enhance overall flexibility, reducing the risk of injury and improving performance in physical activities.

10-Minute Daily Routine
Arm Circles (1 minute)
• Stand up straight and extend your arms to the sides.

Make small circles with your arms, rotating forward for 30 seconds and then backward for another 30 seconds.

Benefit: Warms up shoulder joints, enhances flexibility in the upper body.

Torso Twists (1 minute)
• Stand with your feet shoulder-width apart.

Gently twist your upper body from side to side, feeling the stretch in your waist and spine.

Benefit: Loosens the spine, enhances flexibility in the torso.

Leg Swings (Forward and Backward) (1 minute)

• Hold onto a support for balance.

Swing one leg forward and backward, gradually increasing the range of motion.

Repeat with the other leg.

Benefit: Increases hip mobility, relaxes leg muscles.

Side Bends (1 minute)

• Stand upright, extend one arm overhead, and gently bend sideways.

Alternate sides, feeling the stretch along your side.

Benefit: Stretches side muscles, improves lateral flexibility.

Ankle Bounces (1 minute)

• Stand tall and lightly bounce on the balls of your feet.

Allow your ankles to flex and extend with the bouncing motion.

Benefit: Loosens calf muscles, enhances ankle flexibility.

Shoulder Rolls with Reach (1 minute)

• Roll your shoulders back and down while reaching your arms upward.

Stretch upward, feeling the extension in your shoulders.

Benefit: Stretches shoulder muscles, improves upper body flexibility.

Hip Circles (1 minute)

• Stand with feet hip-width apart and make circular motions with your hips.

Rotate clockwise for 30 seconds and then counterclockwise for another 30 seconds.

Benefit: Increases hip mobility, reduces hip stiffness.

Neck Tilts and Rotations (1 minute)

• Gently tilt your head from side to side and rotate it in circles.

Move slowly and within a comfortable range of motion.

Benefit: Reduces tension in the neck, enhances neck flexibility.

Marching in Place (1 minute)

• Lift your knees up high alternately, as if marching but in one spot. Engage your core and keep a steady pace.

Benefit: Warms up leg muscles, improves circulation.

Full Body Swings (1 minute)

• Stand with feet wider than hip-width apart.

Swing your arms side to side, allowing your torso to follow the movement.

Benefit: Increases overall body flexibility, stretches multiple muscle groups.

**This routine aims to target various muscle groups, improve joint mobility, and enhance overall flexibility within a short duration, providing a comprehensive warm-up for daily activities.

30-Minute Daily Routine

Warm-Up (5 minutes)

• Brisk Walking or Jogging in Place: Start by walking briskly or jogging in place for 5 minutes. This elevates your heart rate and warms up your muscles.

• *Benefit:* Increases blood flow, primes muscles for exercise.

Stretching (5 minutes)

• *Hamstring Stretch*: Sit on the floor, extend one leg forward, lean forward, and reach for your toes. Hold for 20-30 seconds per leg.

• *Quadriceps Stretch*: Stand, bring one foot towards your glutes, hold your ankle, and gently pull your foot toward your body. Hold for 20-30 seconds per leg.

• *Calf Stretch*: Stand near a wall, place one foot behind you, and lean forward, keeping the heel on the ground. Hold for 20-30 seconds per leg.

• *Shoulder Stretch*: Bring one arm across your chest, gently pull it towards your body with the other arm. Hold for 20-30 seconds per arm.

• *Back Stretch*: Sit cross-legged, twist your upper body to one side, using your opposite arm to hug your knee. Hold for 20-30 seconds per side.

Benefits: Enhances flexibility, reduces muscle tension.

Cardiovascular Exercise (10 minutes)

• *Brisk Walking or Cycling*: Engage in brisk walking, cycling, or dancing at a moderate pace for 10 minutes.

Benefit: Boosts heart health and increases endurance.

Strength Training (5 minutes)

• *Bodyweight Squats*: Stand with feet shoulder-width apart, lower into a squat position, then return to standing. Do 2 sets of 10-12 repetitions.

• *Push-Ups*: Begin in a plank position, lower your body, then push back up. Do 2 sets of 10-12 repetitions.

• *Lunges*: Step forward, lower your body until both knees are bent, then return to the starting position. Do 2 sets of 10-12 repetitions per leg.

 Benefit: Builds muscle strength, boosts metabolism.

Core Exercises (5 minutes)

• *Planks*: Hold a plank position on elbows or hands and toes for 30-60 seconds.

• *Russian Twists*: Sit on the floor, lean back slightly, and twist your torso from side to side. Do 2 sets of 10-12 twists per side.

• *Bicycle Crunches*: Lie on your back, bring opposite knee to elbow in a cycling motion. Do 2 sets of 10-12 repetitions per side.

Benefit: Strengthens core muscles, improves stability.

Cool Down and Stretch (5 minutes)

• Slow Walking or Marching in Place: Gradually reduce your pace for 2-3 minutes.

• *Full-Body Stretch*: Stretch major muscle groups: hamstrings, quadriceps, calves, shoulders, and back. Hold each stretch for 20-30 seconds.

Benefit: Prevents muscle soreness, aids in recovery.

**This routine aims to provide a comprehensive workout by incorporating warm-up, stretching, cardiovascular exercise, strength training, core exercises, and a cool-down within a 30-minute time frame.

4

Chapter 4

Upper Body Strength

This chapter aims to equip readers with a range of exercises focusing on the upper body, catering to different abilities and time constraints, while emphasizing safety and effectiveness for seniors.

Seated Arm Exercises
- **Bicep Curls:** Hold a weight in each hand, palms facing forward. Slowly lift the weights towards your shoulders, then lower them back down. Do 2 sets of 10 repetitions. *Benefit*: Strengthens the biceps.

- **Tricep Dips:** Sit at the edge of a sturdy chair, place hands beside hips, fingers facing forward. Slide forward and lower your body by bending elbows, then push back up. Do 2 sets of 10 repetitions.
  Benefit: Targets the triceps.

- **Overhead Press:** Hold a weight in each hand at shoulder height, palms facing forward. Push weights upward until arms are fully extended, then lower back down. Do 2 sets of 10 repetitions.

Benefit: Strengthens shoulders and upper arms.

• **Arm Circles:** Extend arms to the sides at shoulder level. Make small circles forward for 30 seconds, then backward for another 30 seconds.

Benefit: Improves shoulder flexibility and strengthens arm muscles.

• **Shoulder Shrugs:** Hold a weight in each hand, let arms hang by sides. Lift shoulders towards ears, hold for a moment, then lower. Do 2 sets of 15 repetitions.

Benefit: Strengthens and stabilizes shoulder muscles.

• **Wrist Curls:** Hold a weight in each hand, palms facing up. Curl wrists towards your body and then back down. Do 2 sets of 15 repetitions.

Benefit: Strengthens wrists and forearms.

• **Hammer Curls**: Hold a weight in each hand, palms facing your body. Curl weights up toward shoulders, then lower down. Do 2 sets of 10 repetitions.

Benefit: Works both biceps and forearms.

• **Reverse Fly:** Hold weights in each hand, lean forward slightly. Lift arms out to the sides, squeezing shoulder blades together, then lower down. Do 2 sets of 12 repetitions.

Benefit: Targets upper back and rear shoulder muscles.

• **Wrist Extensions:** Hold a weight in each hand, palms facing down. Extend wrists upwards, then lower down. Do 2 sets of 15 repetitions.

Benefit: Strengthens the top part of your forearms.

• **Arm Raises:** Hold a weight in each hand, palms facing thighs. Raise arms forward to shoulder height, then lower back down. Do 2 sets of 12 repetitions.

Benefit: Strengthens shoulder muscles.

**These seated arm exercises target various muscles in the arms, shoulders, and upper back, promoting strength and flexibility while being convenient for seniors or those with mobility limitations.

Wall Push-Up Variations

Standard Wall Push-Up:

• Stand facing a wall, extend your arms at shoulder-width apart, palms flat against the wall.

Lower your body towards the wall by bending your elbows, then push back to the starting position.

Perform 2 sets of 12 repetitions.

Benefit: Strengthens the chest, shoulders, and arms while being a gentle introduction to upper body exercises.

Incline Wall Push-Up:

• Stand a bit farther from the wall than in a standard push-up position.

Place your hands on the wall, wider than shoulder-width apart.

Lower your body towards the wall, maintaining a straight line from head to heels.

Complete 2 sets of 12 repetitions.

Benefit: Engages the chest and shoulders from a different angle, offering a slightly more challenging workout.

One-Leg Wall Push-Up:

• Stand facing the wall, lift one leg off the ground.

Perform a standard or incline wall push-up while balancing on one leg.

Switch legs for each set of 12 repetitions.

Benefit: Enhances balance, engages core muscles, and challenges the upper body simultaneously.

Wide-Arm Wall Push-Up:

• Position hands wider than shoulder-width apart on the wall.

Lower your chest towards the wall, keeping elbows out to the sides.

Push back to the starting position.

Do 2 sets of 12 repetitions.

Benefit: Focuses on the chest muscles and challenges the pectorals differently from standard push-ups.

Decline Wall Push-Up:

• Stand a step or two closer to the wall than in a standard push-up position.

Place your hands on the wall, slightly below shoulder height.

Lower your body towards the wall at an angle, maintaining a straight line from head to heels.

Perform 2 sets of 12 repetitions.

Benefit: Engages the upper chest muscles and shoulders more intensely, providing a higher level of challenge.

**These variations cater to different fitness levels and allow individuals to progress gradually while effectively targeting the upper body muscles, particularly the chest, shoulders, and arms. Adjusting distance, hand placement, or incorporating balance challenges can modulate the exercise intensity.

Resistance Band Techniques
Banded Bicep Curls:

1. Stand on the middle of the band, hold the handles with palms facing up.

2. Curl your hands towards your shoulders, keeping elbows close to your sides.

3. Perform 2 sets of 12 repetitions.

Benefit: Strengthens the biceps, mimicking the movement of traditional bicep curls with weights.

Standing Rows:

1. Step on the band, hold handles, palms facing each other.

2. Pull the band towards your waist, keeping elbows close to your body.

3. Complete 2 sets of 12 repetitions.

Benefit: Targets upper back muscles, improving posture and shoulder stability.

Tricep Extensions:

1. Stand on the band with one foot, hold one handle overhead with both hands.

2. Extend arms upward, then bend at the elbows to lower the band behind your head.

3. Do 2 sets of 12 repetitions.

Benefit: Works the triceps, promoting arm strength and toning.

Front Raises:

1. Stand on the band, hold handles with palms facing down.

2. Lift arms forward to shoulder height, keeping them straight.

3. Perform 2 sets of 12 repetitions.

Benefit: Engages the front shoulder muscles, enhancing shoulder stability.

Lateral Raises:

1. Stand on the band, hold handles with palms facing thighs.

2. Raise arms to the sides at shoulder height, keeping elbows slightly bent.

3. Complete 2 sets of 12 repetitions.

Benefit: Targets side shoulder muscles, improving shoulder strength.

Seated Rows:

1. Sit on the floor, extend legs, loop the band around your feet, hold handles.

2. Pull the band towards your body, squeezing shoulder blades together.

3. Do 2 sets of 12 repetitions.

Benefit: Strengthens the back and shoulders, aiding in posture.

Standing Chest Press:

1. Anchor the band behind you at chest height, hold handles in each hand.

2. Push the handles forward, extending arms in front of you.

3. Perform 2 sets of 12 repetitions.

Benefit: Targets chest muscles, enhancing chest strength.

Band Pull-Aparts:

1. Hold the band in front of you with arms extended, palms facing down.

2. Pull the band apart, bringing hands towards the sides.

3. Complete 2 sets of 12 repetitions.

Benefit: Works rear shoulder muscles, improving posture.

Leg Press:

1. Sit on the floor, loop the band around one foot, hold the other end.

2. Push the foot against the band, straightening the leg.

3. Perform 2 sets of 12 repetitions per leg.

Benefit: Engages leg muscles, specifically quadriceps and hamstrings.

Seated Band Twists:

1. Sit on the floor, hold the band with both hands, arms extended.

2. Rotate your torso from side to side, using the band for resistance.

3. Do 2 sets of 12 repetitions per side.

Benefit: Targets core muscles, promoting core strength and stability.

**These resistance band exercises offer a versatile workout, targeting various muscle groups, promoting strength, and enhancing stability and posture. Adjusting the band tension or the number of repetitions can modify the intensity of the exercises.

Squat Exercise Variations

Bodyweight Squats:

1. Stand with feet shoulder-width apart, toes slightly turned out, hands in front of you or on hips.

2. Lower your body by bending your knees and hips, keeping your chest up and back straight.

3. Descend until thighs are parallel to the floor, then return to standing.

Safety Measure: Keep knees aligned with toes to prevent inward collapsing.

Benefit: Strengthens quads, hamstrings, glutes, and improves overall lower body strength and stability.

Sumo Squats:

1. Widen your stance more than shoulder-width apart, toes pointed

slightly outward.

2. Lower your body into a squat, keeping knees aligned with toes and chest up.

3. Return to the starting position, squeezing the glutes at the top.

Safety Measure: Ensure knees stay in line with toes to avoid strain.

Benefit: Targets inner thighs, glutes, and hamstrings, promoting overall leg strength.

Jump Squats:

1. Begin in a standard squat position, then explode upwards, jumping off the ground.

2. Land softly, returning to the squat position to absorb the impact.

Safety Measure: Land with knees slightly bent to reduce impact on joints.

Benefit: Enhances lower body power, strengthens muscles, and improves explosive strength.

Goblet Squats:

1. Hold a weight or a heavy object close to your chest, elbows pointing down.

2. Lower into a squat, keeping the weight close to the body and chest lifted.

3. Return to standing, maintaining control over the weight.

Safety Measure: Ensure proper weight distribution and control throughout the movement.

Benefit: Targets quads, glutes, and improves core strength and stability.

Single-Leg Squats:

1. Stand on one leg, the other leg extended in front of you.

2. Lower your body by bending the knee of the standing leg, keeping

the extended leg off the ground.

3. Return to standing position without touching the extended leg to the ground.

Safety Measure: Use a support or hold onto a stable object for balance if needed.

Benefit: Enhances balance, strengthens individual leg muscles, and improves stability.

**These squat variations target different muscle groups and offer a range of benefits, from improving strength and stability to boosting explosive power. Adhering to proper form and adjusting the intensity as per individual capabilities is essential for injury prevention and maximizing gains

Single-Leg Stand Variations

Single-Leg Balance:

1. Stand on one leg, keeping the other leg lifted slightly off the ground.
2. Maintain balance for 30 seconds to a minute on each leg.

Safety Measure: Hold onto a stable surface if needed for support.

Benefit: Improves balance, strengthens ankle and lower leg muscles, and enhances stability.

Single-Leg Toe Touch:

1. Stand on one leg, slightly bend the other knee.
2. Slowly hinge at the hips and lower your upper body towards the ground while extending the lifted leg behind you.
3. Reach down toward the floor or as far as comfortable, then return to standing.

Safety Measure: Maintain a slight bend in the supporting knee to avoid locking it.

Benefit: Enhances balance, works on hamstring flexibility, and engages core muscles.

Single-Leg Squat:

1. Balance on one leg, extend the other leg in front.

2. Lower your body into a squat position, keeping the raised leg extended.

3. Return to the starting position.

Safety Measure: Use a stable surface or hold onto an object for balance if needed.

Benefit: Strengthens quadriceps, glutes, and improves stability and balance.

Single-Leg Deadlift:

1. Stand on one leg, slightly bend the knee, keeping a straight back and chest lifted.

2. Hinge at the hips, lowering your torso forward while extending the other leg behind.

3. Keep the back straight and return to a standing position.

Safety Measure: Engage your core and maintain a neutral spine throughout the movement.

Benefit: Targets hamstrings, glutes, and improves balance and hip stability.

Single-Leg Knee Raise:

1. Stand on one leg, raise the opposite knee towards your chest.

2. Hold the position for a few seconds, then lower the leg.

Safety Measure: Keep a stable posture and avoid leaning excessively.

Benefit: Strengthens hip flexors, improves balance, and works on core stability.

**These single legs stand variations focus on improving balance, stability, and strengthening muscles associated with lower body and core strength. Adjusting difficulty levels by holding onto a stable surface or increasing the duration of holds can cater to different fitness levels.

10-Minute Upper Body Routine

• Banded Bicep Curls (2 minutes):

1. Stand on the center of a resistance band, hold handles at shoulder height.

2. Curl your hands towards your shoulders, keeping elbows close to your sides.

Safety Measure: Ensure the band is securely under both feet to prevent slipping.

Benefit: Strengthens biceps, improves arm definition.

Seated Tricep Dips (2 minutes):

1. Sit on a stable chair, place hands beside hips, fingers facing forward.

2. Slide forward off the chair and lower your body by bending elbows, then push back up.

Safety Measure: Ensure the chair is stable and secured.

Benefit: Targets triceps, enhances arm strength and tone.

Resistance Band Rows (2 minutes):

1. Anchor the band at waist height, hold handles, step back to create tension.

2. Pull the band towards your waist, squeezing shoulder blades together.

Safety Measure: Maintain proper posture to avoid straining the lower back.

Benefit: Works upper back muscles, improves posture.

Overhead Press with Weights (2 minutes):

1. Hold weights at shoulder height, palms facing forward.

2. Push weights upward until arms are fully extended, then lower back down.

Safety Measure: Use appropriate weights to prevent strain.

Benefit: Strengthens shoulders, tones deltoids.

Front Plank (2 minutes):

1. Assume a plank position on elbows and toes, keeping the body straight.

2. Engage core muscles and hold the position.

Safety Measure: Maintain a straight line from head to heels, avoid arching or sagging.

Benefit: Engages core muscles, improves overall stability.

**These routines target major upper body muscle groups, including arms, shoulders, back, and core. Adjusting band tension or weights according to your fitness level is crucial for effective and safe workouts. Incorporating this routine regularly can lead to improved upper body strength and toning.

30-Minute Upper Body Routine

Warm-up (3 minutes):

Arm Circles: Stand tall, extend arms to the sides, and make circular motions forward and backward for 1 minute each.

Benefits: Increases blood flow, prepares muscles for the workout.

Banded Bicep Curls (4 minutes):

Stand on the center of a resistance band, hold handles at shoulder height.

Curl your hands towards your shoulders, keeping elbows close to your sides.

Safety Measure: Ensure proper band placement for stability.

Benefit: Strengthens biceps, tones arms.

Triceps Kickbacks (4 minutes):

Hold a weight in each hand, hinge forward at the hips with a flat back.

Extend arms behind, then bend at the elbows to return to the starting position.

Safety Measure: Maintain a neutral spine and avoid using excessive weight.

Benefit: Targets triceps, enhances arm definition.

Resistance Band Rows (4 minutes):

Anchor the band at waist height, hold handles, step back to create tension.

Pull the band towards your waist, squeezing shoulder blades together.

Safety Measure: Ensure proper band tension and form.

Benefit: Works upper back muscles, improves posture.

Overhead Press with Weights (4 minutes):

Hold weights at shoulder height, palms facing forward.

Push weights upward until arms are fully extended, then lower back down.

Safety Measure: Use appropriate weights and maintain proper form.

Benefit: Strengthens shoulders, tones deltoids.

Chest Press with Weights (4 minutes):

Lie on your back, hold weights above the chest, elbows bent.

Push weights upward until arms are straight, then lower back down.

Safety Measure: Ensure a stable position and controlled movements.

Benefit: Targets chest muscles, improves chest strength.

Plank Variations (4 minutes):

Forearm Plank: Hold a plank position on elbows and toes for 2 minutes.

Side Plank (Each Side): Balance on one forearm and the side of the foot for 1 minute each side.

Safety Measure: Maintain a straight line from head to heels in all plank variations.

Benefit: Engages core muscles, improves stability.

Cool-down and Stretch (4 minutes):

Shoulder Stretch: Hold each shoulder stretch for 30 seconds.

Arm Across Chest Stretch: Hold each arm stretch for 30 seconds.

Benefits: Reduces muscle tension, increases flexibility.

**These routine targets various upper body muscle groups while also incorporating warm-up, strength, and cool-down phases.

***Adhering to proper form, using suitable weights, and focusing on controlled movements are essential for safety and effectiveness.

5

Chapter 5

Importance of Core Strengthening and Its Benefits

Why Core Strengthening Matters:

A strong core is the foundation for stability and movement in the body. The core comprises muscles in the abdomen, lower back, pelvis, and hips, essential for supporting the spine and maintaining proper posture. Strengthening these muscles plays a pivotal role in everyday activities, from simple tasks to complex movements.

Benefits of Core Strengthening:

1. **Improved Posture**: A strong core helps maintain proper alignment, reducing strain on the spine and enhancing posture.

2. **Enhanced Stability and Balance**: Core strength contributes to better balance, reducing the risk of falls and injuries, especially in older adults.

3. **Reduced Back Pain:** Strengthening core muscles can alleviate lower back pain by providing better support to the spine and reducing stress on the back.

4. **Enhanced Athletic Performance:** A strong core is crucial for

athletes, improving performance in various sports and activities by providing a stable base for movement.

5. **Functional Strength:** Core strength is fundamental for everyday tasks like lifting, bending, and twisting, making these movements easier and safer.

6. **Injury Prevention:** A robust core can prevent injuries by supporting proper movement patterns and reducing stress on other body parts.

7. **Improved Breathing and Digestion**: Strengthening core muscles can aid in better breathing mechanics and support proper digestion.

8. **Enhanced Overall Fitness**: A strong core complements overall fitness, allowing for better performance in other workouts and activities.

By understanding the significance of core strengthening and the multitude of benefits it offers, we can focus on exercises that specifically target these crucial muscle groups, promoting overall health and well-being. By highlighting the importance and advantages of core strengthening, I am hoping to encourage you to choose to prioritize exercises that enhance core stability and strength for better overall health and functionality.

Seated Core Exercises

Seated Russian Twists:

1. Sit on the floor with knees bent, heels on the ground, lean back slightly, and clasp hands together.

2. Twist your torso to the right, bringing your hands close to the ground beside your hip, then twist to the left.

3. Perform 3 sets of 12 twists on each side.

Benefit: Engages obliques, strengthens core stability.

Seated Knee Tucks:

1. Sit on the edge of a chair, hold the sides for support, lean back slightly, and lift your knees towards your chest.

2. Extend legs outward, then pull knees back in.

3. Do 3 sets of 15 knee tucks.

Benefit: Works on lower abdominals, improves core strength.

Seated Leg Raises:

1. Sit on a chair, keep your back straight, and hold onto the sides of the chair for support.

2. Lift both legs straight out in front of you, then lower them back down without touching the floor.

3. Perform 3 sets of 12 leg raises.

Benefit: Targets lower abdominal muscles, enhances core stability.

Seated Bicycle Crunches:

1. Sit on a chair, place hands behind your head, and lift your legs off the ground slightly.

2. Bring the right elbow towards the left knee while extending the right leg forward, then alternate sides.

3. Complete 3 sets of 15 bicycle crunches on each side.

Benefit: Engages the entire core, improves core endurance.

Seated Toe Touches:

1. Sit on a chair, straighten your legs in front of you.

2. Reach forward, aiming to touch your toes while keeping legs straight, then return to the starting position.

3. Perform 3 sets of 12 toe touches.

Benefit: Stretches and strengthens abdominal muscles.

Pelvic Floor Activation Exercises

Kegels:

1. Sit or lie comfortably, contract the pelvic floor muscles as if

stopping urine flow.

2. Hold for 5 seconds, then relax. Repeat 10-15 times.

Benefit: Strengthens pelvic floor muscles, aids in bladder control.

Bridge:

1. Lie on your back with knees bent, feet flat on the floor.

2. Lift your hips off the ground, squeezing glutes and engaging pelvic floor muscles.

3. Hold for 5-10 seconds, then lower. Repeat 10 times.

Benefit: Strengthens pelvic muscles, improves core stability.

Squats:

1. Stand with feet hip-width apart, squat down as if sitting back into a chair.

2. Engage pelvic floor muscles while squatting and return to standing.

3. Do 3 sets of 10 squats.

Benefit: Works on pelvic muscle strength and stability.

Supine Abdominal Breathing:

1. Lie on your back, place hands on your abdomen.

2. Inhale deeply, expanding the abdomen, then exhale, drawing the navel in towards the spine.

3. Repeat for 10 breaths.

Benefit: Enhances pelvic floor coordination with breathing.

Pilates Hundred:

1. Lie on your back, legs lifted, arms reaching forward.

2. Pump your arms up and down while engaging core and pelvic muscles.

3. Do 5 sets of 10 arm pumps.

Benefit: Engages core and pelvic floor muscles.

Wall Squats with Ball Squeeze:

1. Place a small ball between knees against a wall.

2. Perform squats while squeezing the ball, engaging inner thighs and pelvic floor.

3. Do 3 sets of 12 squats.

Benefit: Strengthens pelvic floor and inner thigh muscles.

Leg Slides:

1. Lie on your back, knees bent, feet flat on the floor.

2. Slide one leg out, engaging the pelvic floor, then return to the starting position.

3. Alternate legs for 10 reps on each side.

Benefit: Activates pelvic floor while working hip mobility.

Standing Pelvic Tilts:

1. Stand with feet shoulder-width apart, engage core muscles.

2. Tilt pelvis forward and backward, contracting and releasing pelvic floor muscles.

3. Perform 15-20 tilts.

Benefit: Helps in pelvic floor muscle control.

Butterfly Stretch:

1. Sit on the floor, soles of feet together, knees bent outwards.

2. Gently press knees towards the floor, engaging pelvic floor muscles.

3. Hold the stretch for 30 seconds, repeat 3 times.

Benefit: Stretches and strengthens pelvic floor muscles.

Belly Breathing:

1. Lie on your back, place your hands on your belly.

2. Inhale deeply, expanding the abdomen, then exhale, engaging pelvic floor muscles.

3. Repeat for 10 breaths.

Benefit: Helps coordinate breathing and pelvic muscle engagement.

**Performing these pelvic floor activation exercises regularly can enhance pelvic floor strength, improve control, and support overall core stability.

***Adjust repetitions and intensity according to your comfort and fitness level.

Modified Planks for Pelvic Activation

Incline Plank:

1. Begin in a standing position, leaning against a sturdy surface like a countertop or wall.

2. Place hands on the surface, slightly wider than shoulder-width apart, and step feet back.

3. Keep the body straight from head to heels, engaging the core and pelvic muscles.

4. Hold the position for 20-30 seconds, gradually increasing duration.

Safety Measure: Maintain a neutral spine, avoid arching or sagging.

Benefit: Activates core and pelvic muscles with less stress on wrists and shoulders.

Forearm Plank on Knees:

1. Start on all fours, lower onto forearms, ensuring elbows are under shoulders.

2. Extend legs backward, resting on knees instead of toes, keeping the body straight.

3. Engage core and pelvic muscles, hold for 20-30 seconds.

4. Safety Measure: Keep the back flat and avoid overarching.

Benefit: Aids in pelvic activation with reduced strain on lower back.

Side Plank with Knee Support:

1. Begin in a side plank position on your forearm, keeping knees bent and resting on the lower knee.

2. Raise hips, forming a straight line from head to knees, engaging core and pelvic muscles.

3. Hold for 15-20 seconds, then switch sides.

Safety Measure: Ensure the hips are lifted to maintain alignment.

Benefit: Targets pelvic muscles while offering additional stability.

Plank with Leg Lifts:

1. Assume a standard plank position on forearms and toes, maintaining a straight line.

2. Lift one leg a few inches off the ground while engaging the core and pelvic muscles.

3. Alternate legs for 10 lifts on each side.

Safety Measure: Avoid excessive hip rotation or lifting.

Benefit: Engages pelvic muscles and improves stability.

Elevated Plank on Bench or Chair:

1. Position forearms on an elevated surface (like a bench or chair), legs extended behind.

2. Maintain a straight line from head to heels, engaging core and pelvic muscles.

3. Hold for 20-30 seconds, focusing on stability.

Safety Measure: Ensure a stable surface and proper forearm placement.

Benefit: Challenges pelvic activation while adjusting intensity.

**These modified plank variations offer different levels of intensity and support for pelvic activation, ensuring proper engagement of core and pelvic muscles while minimizing strain on other parts of the body.

***As with any exercise, maintaining proper form and gradual progression is key to safety and effectiveness.

10-Minute Daily Core Strengthening Routine

Warm-up: Begin with 1-2 minutes of light walking or marching in place to prepare the body for exercise.

Seated Marches (1 minute):

1. Sit on a chair with feet flat on the floor.

2. Lift one foot slightly off the ground and alternate with the other foot, as if marching.

3. Engage core muscles during the movement.

Benefit: Activates core and improves hip flexibility.

Seated Russian Twists (1 minute):

1. Sit on a chair with knees bent and feet flat.

2. Clasp hands together and twist your torso from side to side.

3. Engage core and pelvic muscles while twisting.

Benefit: Works on oblique muscles and enhances core stability.

Seated Knee Tucks (1 minute):

1. Sit on the edge of a chair, hold the sides for support.

2. Lean back slightly and lift your knees towards your chest.

3. Alternate extending legs outward, then pulling knees back in.

Benefit: Strengthens lower abdominal muscles and improves core strength.

Bridge (1 minute):

1. Lie on your back with knees bent, feet flat on the floor.

2. Lift your hips off the ground, squeezing glutes and engaging pelvic floor muscles.

3. Hold for a few seconds, then lower back down.

Benefit: Engages core and improves lower back strength.

Pelvic Tilts (1 minute):

1. Sit on a chair with feet flat, hands on hips.
2. Tilt the pelvis forward and backward, contracting and releasing pelvic muscles.
3. Perform controlled movements.

Benefit: Strengthens and stabilizes pelvic floor muscles.

Plank with Knee Support (2 minutes):

1. Begin on all fours, lower onto forearms, ensuring elbows are under shoulders.
2. Extend legs backward, resting on knees instead of toes, keeping the body straight.
3. Engage core and pelvic muscles, holding the position.

Benefit: Aids in pelvic activation and core stability.

Cool-down: Finish with 1-2 minutes of slow walking or stretching to ease muscles.

**This routine incorporates seated and modified exercises suitable for seniors, focusing on core activation and stability. Prioritize maintaining proper form and breathing throughout the routine.

***Adjust repetitions or rest as needed and gradually increase intensity over time. Always consult a healthcare professional before starting any new exercise routine.

30-Minute Daily Core Strengthening Routine

Warm-up: Begin with 2-3 minutes of light walking or marching in place to prepare the body for exercise.

Seated Marches (3 minutes):

1. Sit on a chair with feet flat on the floor.

2. Lift one foot slightly off the ground and alternate with the other foot, as if marching.

3. Engage core muscles during the movement.

Benefit: Activates core and improves hip flexibility.

Seated Russian Twists (3 minutes):

1. Sit on a chair with knees bent and feet flat.

2. Clasp hands together and twist your torso from side to side.

3. Engage core and pelvic muscles while twisting.

Benefit: Works on oblique muscles and enhances core stability.

Seated Knee Tucks (3 minutes):

1. Sit on the edge of a chair, hold the sides for support.

2. Lean back slightly and lift your knees towards your chest.

3. Alternate extending legs outward, then pulling knees back in.

Benefit: Strengthens lower abdominal muscles and improves core strength.

Bridge (3 minutes):

1. Lie on your back with knees bent, feet flat on the floor.

2. Lift your hips off the ground, squeezing glutes and engaging pelvic floor muscles.

3. Hold for a few seconds, then lower back down.

Benefit: Engages core and improves lower back strength.

Pelvic Tilts (3 minutes):

1. Sit on a chair with feet flat, hands on hips.

2. Tilt the pelvis forward and backward, contracting and releasing pelvic muscles.

3. Perform controlled movements.

Benefit: Strengthens and stabilizes pelvic floor muscles.

Plank with Knee Support (5 minutes):

1. Begin on all fours, lower onto forearms, ensuring elbows are under shoulders.

2. Extend legs backward, resting on knees instead of toes, keeping the body straight.

3. Engage core and pelvic muscles, holding the position.

Benefit: Aids in pelvic activation and core stability.

Side Planks with Knee Support (5 minutes):

1. Begin in a side plank position on your forearm, keeping knees bent and resting on the lower knee.

2. Raise hips, forming a straight line from head to knees, engaging core and pelvic muscles.

3. Hold for 30 seconds, then switch sides.

Benefit: Targets pelvic muscles while offering additional stability.

Cool-down: Finish with 3-5 minutes of gentle stretching for the entire body, focusing on the core, hips, and lower back.

**This routine focuses on seated and modified exercises suitable for seniors, emphasizing core activation, stability, and strength. Ensure proper form and breathing throughout the routine.

***Adjust repetitions, rest, or modify exercises as needed and gradually increase intensity over time. Always consult a healthcare professional before starting any new exercise routine.

6

Chapter 6

Lower Body Strength

This section will focus on exercises to strengthen the lower body, enhancing stability and mobility.

Chair-Based Squats

Standard Chair Squat:

1. Stand in front of a chair with feet shoulder-width apart.

2. Lower yourself toward the chair as if about to sit, then stand back up.

Benefit: Strengthens quadriceps, hamstrings, and glutes.

Single Leg Squat to Chair:

1. Stand on one leg in front of the chair, keeping the other leg lifted.

2. Lower yourself toward the chair with control, then return to standing.

Benefit: Enhances balance and strengthens legs individually.

Sumo Squats with Chair:

1. Stand with feet wider than shoulder-width apart, toes pointing outwards.

2. Lower into a squat, aiming to touch the chair, then return to standing.

Benefit: Targets inner thighs and glutes.

Pulse Squats:

1. Stand in front of the chair and lower into a squat position.

2. Perform tiny pulses up and down without fully standing up.

Benefit: Engages leg muscles more intensely.

Split Squats:

1. Stand facing away from the chair, one foot elevated on the seat.

2. Lower the back knee toward the floor, then push back up.

Benefit: Works on quadriceps and glutes of the front leg.

Isometric Chair Squat:

1. Lower into a squat position and hold it without sitting.

2. Maintain the position for a specific duration.

Benefit: Builds strength and endurance in leg muscles.

Side-to-Side Squats:

1. Stand next to the chair with feet together.

2. Step one foot to the side into a squat, then return to center and repeat on the other side.

Benefit: Engages inner and outer thigh muscles.

Chair Tap Squats:

1. Stand in front of the chair, then squat down and lightly tap the chair with your bottom.

2. Push back up to standing without sitting.

Benefit: Reinforces proper squat depth and control.

Eccentric Squats:

1. Start standing, then slowly lower into a squat, taking a count of 3-5 seconds.

2. Stand back up to the starting position.

Benefit: Focuses on muscle control and strength during the lowering phase.

**These chair-based squat variations offer a range of intensities and target different muscle groups within the lower body, contributing to improved strength, stability, and overall mobility.

***Always prioritize proper form and consult with a healthcare professional before starting any new exercise routine.

Leg Raises and Extensions

Seated Knee Extensions:

1. Sit on the edge of a chair, extend one leg forward, hold briefly, then lower.

2. Alternate legs, aiming for 10-15 repetitions on each side.

Benefit: Strengthens quadriceps and improves knee stability.

Seated Leg Raises:

1. Sit tall in the chair with feet hovering slightly above the ground.

2. Lift both legs straight out in front, hold for a few seconds, then lower.

3. Aim for 10-12 repetitions.

Benefit: Targets abdominal muscles and enhances hip flexor strength.

Standing Leg Extensions:

1. Hold onto the back of a chair for support, stand tall with feet

hip-width apart.

2.   Extend one leg backward, keeping it straight, then return to standing position.

3. Perform 10-12 repetitions on each leg.

Benefit: Works on hamstring muscles and improves balance.

Seated Bicycle Kicks:

1. Sit comfortably on the chair, lean back slightly, and lift legs off the ground.

2. Pedal your legs as if riding a bicycle, bringing knees towards chest alternatively.

3. Do this for 30-60 seconds.

Benefit: Engages abdominal muscles and enhances core stability.

Seated Leg Circles:

1. Sit on the chair with legs extended, and draw circles with your toes.

2. Rotate clockwise for 10 circles, then switch to counterclockwise.

Benefit: Boosts hip flexibility and strengthens hip abductors.

Standing Side Leg Lifts:

1. Stand behind the chair, hold onto it for balance.

2. Lift one leg out to the side, keeping it straight, then lower.

3. Complete 10-12 reps on each leg.

Benefit: Targets outer thigh muscles and enhances hip strength.

Seated Heel Taps:

1. Sit on the chair, feet flat on the ground.

2. Lift one foot slightly off the ground and tap the heel in front of you.

3. Alternate between legs for 10-12 repetitions on each side.

Benefit: Works on quadriceps and calf muscles.

Seated Inner Thigh Squeezes:

1. Sit on the chair with a soft ball or cushion between your knees.

2. Squeeze the ball with your inner thighs, hold for a few seconds, then release.

3. Repeat for 12-15 squeezes.

Benefit: Strengthens inner thigh muscles and improves hip stability.

Seated Leg Crosses:

1. Sit tall in the chair with legs extended and crossed at the ankles.

2. Alternate crossing one leg over the other, then switch sides.

3. Perform 10-12 crosses on each side.

Benefit: Engages outer thigh muscles and improves hip flexibility.

Seated Calf Raises:

1. Sit with feet flat on the floor, lift heels off the ground as high as possible.

2. Lower heels back down and repeat for 12-15 repetitions.

Benefit: Targets calf muscles and aids in ankle stability.

**These leg raise and extension exercises are varied and target different muscles within the legs and core, contributing to improved strength, flexibility, and balance.

***Always maintain proper form and consult with a healthcare professional before starting any new exercise routine.

Heel Toe Raises

Seated Heel Raises:

1. Sit in a chair with feet flat on the ground.

2. Lift your heels as high as possible while keeping the balls of your feet grounded.

3. Slowly lower heels back down.

Benefit: Strengthens calf muscles and improves ankle mobility.

Seated Toe Raises:

1. Sit in a chair with heels on the ground and toes lifted upward.

2. Lower toes back down and repeat the movement.

Benefit: Works on shin muscles and helps prevent shin splints.

Standing Heel Raises:

1. Stand tall behind a chair or counter for support.

2. Rise onto the balls of your feet, lifting heels off the ground.

3. Lower heels back down slowly.

Benefit: Strengthens calf muscles and enhances balance.

Standing Toe Raises:

1. Stand tall and lift your toes upward while keeping heels grounded.

2. Lower toes back down and repeat.

Benefit: Engages muscles on the front of the lower leg.

Heel Walking:

1. Lift toes off the ground, walk on heels for a short distance.

2. Maintain balance and control while walking.

Benefit: Strengthens calf muscles and improves ankle stability.

Toe Walking:

1. Lift heels off the ground, walk on toes for a short distance.

2. Focus on balance and maintaining an upright posture.

Benefit: Works on muscles in the front of the lower leg and enhances balance.

Seated Heel-to-Toe Taps:
1. Sit on a chair with feet flat on the floor.
2. Tap your toes and heels alternately on the ground.
Benefit: Enhances foot and ankle flexibility.

Balancing on Toes:
1. Stand behind a chair or counter for support.
2. Rise onto the balls of your feet and hold the position for 10-15 seconds.
Benefit: Improves calf strength and balance.

Balancing on Heels:
1. Stand behind a chair or counter for support.
2. Lift toes off the ground and balance on the heels for 10-15 seconds.
Benefit: Works on ankle stability and calf muscles.

Ankle Alphabet:
1. Sit in a chair, lift one foot off the ground, and write the alphabet with your toes.
2. Repeat with the other foot.
Benefit: Improves ankle mobility and strengthens toe muscles.
**These heel toe raise exercises offer diverse movements to target different muscles in the feet, ankles, and lower legs, promoting strength, flexibility, and improved balance.
***Always maintain proper form and consult with a healthcare professional before starting any new exercise routine.

Chair-Based Circuit Training

Seated Marches:

1. Sit on the edge of the chair, lift knees up one at a time, mimicking a marching motion.

2. Perform for 1 minute.

Benefit: Engages core muscles and improves cardiovascular endurance.

Chair Dips:

1. Sit on the edge of the chair, grip the seat's edge with hands, slide off the chair, and lower yourself downward.

2. Push back up to the starting position.

Benefit: Strengthens triceps and shoulders.

Seated Knee Extensions:

1. Sit tall in the chair, extend one leg forward, hold briefly, and return to the starting position.

2. Alternate legs for 10 repetitions on each side.

Benefit: Targets quadriceps and enhances knee stability.

Seated Side Leg Lifts:

1. Sit upright, slightly away from the backrest, and lift one leg out to the side.

2. Lower the leg and repeat on the other side.

3. Do 10-12 lifts on each side.

Benefit: Strengthens outer thigh muscles and improves hip stability.

Seated Torso Twists:

1. Sit tall, hold a ball or light weight, rotate your torso to one side, then the other.

2. Perform 10 twists on each side.

Benefit: Engages oblique muscles and enhances spinal mobility.

Seated Leg Circles:

1. Sit with feet slightly off the ground, draw circles with toes.

2. Rotate clockwise for 10 circles, then switch to counterclockwise.

Benefit: Boosts hip flexibility and strengthens leg muscles.

Seated Toe Taps:

1. Sit tall, tap toes lightly on the ground alternately.

2. Increase speed for 30 seconds.

Benefit: Enhances circulation and foot flexibility.

Seated Arm Circles:

1. Sit tall, extend arms to the sides, and make circular motions with your arms.

2. Perform 10 circles forward, then 10 circles backward.

Benefit: Warms up shoulder muscles and improves mobility.

Seated High Knees:

1. Sit upright, lift knees toward the chest alternately, engaging core muscles.

2. Perform for 1 minute.

Benefit: Boosts heart rate and works on lower abdominal muscles.

Seated Leg Press:

1. Sit with feet flat on the floor, press both feet against the chair's base, then release.

2. Repeat for 10-12 reps.

Benefit: Targets quadriceps and calf muscles.

**These chair-based circuit training exercises offer a comprehensive workout, engaging various muscle groups and promoting overall strength, flexibility, and cardiovascular fitness.

***Always prioritize proper form and consult with a healthcare professional before starting any new exercise routine.

10-Minute Daily Routine for Lower Body Strength

Chair Squats (1 minute):

Stand in front of a chair, lower your body as if sitting down, then return to standing.

Benefit: Strengthens quadriceps, hamstrings, and glutes; improves lower body strength.

Leg Raises (1 minute):

Stand behind a chair for support, lift one leg backward, then lower it.

Benefit: Targets glutes and hamstrings; enhances hip stability.

Heel Raises (1 minute):

Stand tall, raise onto your toes, then lower back down.

Benefit: Strengthens calf muscles and improves ankle stability.

Side Leg Raises (1 minute):

Stand next to a chair, lift one leg sideways, then lower it.

Benefit: Engages outer thigh muscles; enhances hip flexibility.

Wall Sit (1 minute):

Lean against a wall, slide down until thighs are parallel to the ground, hold the position.

Benefit: Strengthens quadriceps, hamstrings, and glutes; improves lower body endurance.

Standing Calf Raises (1 minute):

Stand tall, lift onto the balls of your feet, then lower heels back down.

Benefit: Targets calf muscles; improves ankle strength.

Forward Lunges (1 minute):

Take a step forward, lower your body until both knees form 90-degree angles, then return to standing.

Benefit: Works quadriceps, hamstrings, and glutes; enhances balance.

Backward Leg Raises (1 minute):

Hold onto a chair, lift one leg backward, then lower it.

Benefit: Engages glutes and hamstrings; enhances hip stability.

Toe Taps (1 minute):

Stand, tap one foot backward, then return to the starting position, alternate legs.

Benefit: Targets lower body muscles; improves coordination.

Step-Ups (1 minute):

Use a stable step or platform, step up with one foot, then step down and alternate legs.

Benefit: Strengthens lower body muscles; enhances balance and coordination.

**This routine offers a range of lower body strength exercises suitable for senior adults, focusing on various muscle groups while promoting stability and mobility. ***Always maintain proper form, listen to your body, and consult with a healthcare professional before starting any new exercise routine.

30-Minute Daily Routine for Lower Body Strength
Warm-Up (5 minutes)

• Begin with light marching in place or walking to warm up the muscles and increase heart rate.

Lower Body Exercises (25 minutes)

Seated Leg Press (3 minutes):

• Sit in a chair, press both feet against the chair's base, then release.

Benefit: Targets quadriceps and calf muscles; improves leg strength.

Standing Hip Abduction (3 minutes):

• Stand near a chair, lift one leg sideways, then return to the starting position.

Benefit: Engages hip abductor muscles; improves hip stability.

Box Squats (3 minutes):

• Use a sturdy box or chair, sit down, then stand back up.

Benefit: Strengthens quadriceps, hamstrings, and glutes; enhances lower body strength.

Heel-to-Toe Walk (3 minutes):

• Walk in a straight line, placing the heel of one foot directly in front of the toes of the other foot.

Benefit: Enhances balance and stability; engages lower leg muscles.

Standing Calf Stretch (3 minutes):

• Stand facing a wall, place hands against it, step one foot back, press the heel down.

Benefit: Stretches calf muscles; improves flexibility and prevents tightness.

Bridge Exercise (3 minutes):

• Lie on your back, knees bent, lift hips off the ground, hold briefly, then lower.

Benefit: Strengthens glutes, hamstrings, and lower back; improves hip stability.

Side Step-Ups (3 minutes):

• Use a step or platform, step sideways onto it, then step down and alternate legs.

Benefit: Works outer thigh muscles; enhances balance and coordination.

Standing Hip Extension (3 minutes):

• Stand holding onto a chair, lift one leg backward, then return to the starting position.

Benefit: Engages glutes and hamstrings; improves hip mobility.

Lateral Leg Raises (3 minutes):

• Stand tall, lift one leg sideways, then lower it; alternate legs.

Benefit: Targets outer thigh muscles; improves hip stability.

Cool Down (5 minutes)

• Conclude with gentle stretches focusing on the lower body muscles, holding each stretch for about 30 seconds.

**This routine offers a comprehensive set of lower body exercises for senior adults, focusing on strength, stability, and flexibility.

***Prioritize proper form, listen to your body, and consult with a healthcare professional before starting any new exercise routine.

7

Chapter 7

Flexibility and Balance

This chapter is structured to introduce exercises catering to flexibility and balance, offering readers a range of routines and practices suitable for their daily schedules and aimed at enhancing their overall mobility and stability.

Seated and Standing Stretches
for Flexibility and Balance

Seated Forward Fold:

· Sit on a chair, hinge at your hips, and reach forward towards your toes. Hold for 15-30 seconds.

Benefit: Stretches the hamstrings, lower back, and improves flexibility in the spine.

Standing Quadriceps Stretch:

· Stand next to a chair, grab one ankle and gently pull towards your buttocks. Hold for 15-30 seconds per leg.

Benefit: Stretches the front of the thigh, improves balance, and flexibility.

Side Stretch:

· Sit or stand, raise one arm overhead, lean sideways to the opposite direction. Hold for 15-30 seconds each side.

Benefit: Stretches the sides of the torso, promoting flexibility and better range of motion.

Seated Spinal Twist:

· Sit tall, twist your upper body to one side while holding onto the back of the chair. Hold for 15-30 seconds each side.

Benefit: Stretches the spine, improves flexibility and spinal mobility.

Standing Calf Stretch:

· Stand near a wall, place both hands on the wall, step one foot back and press the heel into the ground. Hold for 15-30 seconds per leg.

Benefit: Stretches calf muscles, improves ankle flexibility and prevents tightness.

Seated Hip Stretch:

· Sit on the edge of a chair, cross one ankle over the opposite knee, gently press the crossed knee down. Hold for 15-30 seconds per side.

Benefit: Stretches the hip muscles, improves flexibility, and eases hip tension.

Standing Hamstring Stretch:

· Stand tall, extend one leg forward with toes pointed up, lean forward from your hips. Hold for 15-30 seconds per leg.

Benefit: Stretches the hamstrings, improves flexibility in the back of the leg.

Seated Shoulder Stretch:

· Sit tall, reach one arm across your chest, use the opposite hand to gently press the arm closer. Hold for 15-30 seconds each side.

Benefit: Stretches the shoulders and upper back, enhances upper body flexibility.

Standing Inner Thigh Stretch:

· Stand with legs wide apart, shift your weight to one side, lean towards the bent leg. Hold for 15-30 seconds per side.

Benefit: Stretches inner thigh muscles, improves groin flexibility.

Seated Neck Stretch:

· Sit tall, gently tilt your head to one side, allowing your ear to approach the shoulder. Hold for 15-30 seconds each side.

Benefit: Relieves neck tension, improves neck flexibility and range of motion.

**These exercises offer a combination of seated and standing stretches targeting various muscle groups, promoting flexibility, and aiding in better balance and mobility.

***Always perform stretches gently and avoid any movements causing discomfort or pain.

**Tai Chi-Inspired Movements for Flexibility and Balance
Weight Shifting:**

· Stand with feet shoulder-width apart, gently shift weight from one leg to the other in a slow, controlled manner.

Benefit: Enhances balance, strengthens leg muscles, and promotes stability.

Cloud Hands:

· Stand with knees slightly bent, arms extended to the sides. Rotate your torso gently from side to side in a flowing motion.

Benefit: Increases flexibility in the spine, improves coordination, and balance.

Wave Hands Like Clouds:

· Stand with feet shoulder-width apart, shift weight to one leg while circling both arms in front of you, then switch sides.

Benefit: Enhances upper body flexibility, strengthens core muscles, and improves balance.

Grasp Sparrow's Tail:

· Stand tall, step forward with one foot, raise your arms in front of you, then sweep them to the sides while shifting weight back.

Benefit: Improves leg strength, enhances flexibility, and balance in lower body muscles.

Parting the Wild Horse's Mane:

· Stand with feet shoulder-width apart, step to the side and shift weight onto that leg while extending one arm forward and the other back.

Benefit: Strengthens leg muscles, improves hip flexibility, and balance.

White Crane Spreads its Wings:

· Stand with feet shoulder-width apart, lift one knee while raising both arms overhead, then switch legs.

Benefit: Enhances balance, strengthens leg muscles, and improves overall flexibility.

Brush Knee and Twist Step:

· Stand with feet shoulder-width apart, step forward, and twist your torso while shifting weight between legs.

Benefit Improves lower body flexibility, strengthens leg muscles, and enhances balance.

Repulse Monkey:

· Stand with feet shoulder-width apart, step back while extending one arm forward, then shift weight and switch arms.

Benefit: Increases flexibility in the shoulders, strengthens leg muscles, and improves balance.

Waving Hands in Clouds:

· Stand with feet shoulder-width apart, gently sway your arms in a circular motion while shifting weight from side to side.

Benefit: Enhances coordination, flexibility in the arms and shoulders, and promotes overall balance.

Golden Rooster Stands on One Leg:

· Stand tall, shift weight to one leg, and raise the opposite knee while balancing on one leg.

Benefit Improves leg strength, stability, and overall balance.

**These Tai Chi-inspired movements prioritize slow, deliberate motions to enhance flexibility, balance, and coordination. Incorporating these exercises can promote overall physical well-being and help reduce the risk of falls.

Yoga for Seniors: Flexibility and Balance

Mountain Pose (Tadasana):

· Stand tall, feet together or hip-width apart, arms relaxed by your sides. Engage core muscles, elongate the spine, and breathe deeply.

Benefit: Enhances posture, strengthens legs and feet, improves balance and concentration.

Tree Pose (Vrikshasana):

· Stand with feet grounded, shift weight to one leg, place the sole of the other foot on the inner thigh or calf, hands at heart center or overhead.

Benefits: Improves balance, strengthens leg muscles, and enhances concentration.

Chair Pose (Utkatasana):

· Stand with feet together, bend knees as if sitting back into an imaginary chair, raise arms parallel to the floor or overhead.

Benefit: Strengthens thighs, calves, and back muscles, improves balance and endurance.

Warrior II (Virabhadrasana II):

· Stand with legs wide apart, turn one foot out, bend the front knee, extend arms parallel to the floor, gaze over the front hand.

Benefit: Stretches hips and groin, strengthens legs, improves balance, and focus.

Seated Forward Fold (Paschimottanasana):

· Sit on a chair or floor, extend legs forward, hinge at the hips, reach for toes or shins, keeping the spine lengthened.

Benefit: Stretches hamstrings and lower back, enhances spine flexibility, and reduces stress.

Cat-Cow Stretch (Marjaryasana-Bitilasana):

· Begin on hands and knees, arch your back upward like a cat (cow pose) and then drop the belly down while lifting the head (cow pose).

Benefit: Improves spinal flexibility, strengthens back muscles, and massages organs.

Seated Spinal Twist:

· Sit tall on a chair or the floor, twist the torso to one side, hold onto the chair's arm or knee, and gaze over the shoulder.

Benefit: Stretches the spine, hips, and shoulders, improves spinal mobility and digestion.

Bridge Pose (Setu Bandhasana):

· Lie on your back, bend knees, feet flat on the floor, lift hips upward, interlace fingers under your back, and press shoulders into the floor.

Benefit: Strengthens back, buttocks, and hamstrings, stretches chest, and improves spine flexibility.

Legs-Up-the-Wall (Viparita Karani):

· Lie on the floor near a wall, extend legs upward against the wall, arms by the sides or on the belly.

Benefit: Reduces swelling in the legs, relaxes lower back, promotes relaxation, and improves circulation.

Corpse Pose (Savasana):

· Lie on your back, arms at your sides, legs comfortably apart, close your eyes, and focus on deep breathing.

Benefit: Promotes relaxation, reduces stress, and allows the body to absorb the benefits of the practice.

**These yoga exercises cater to seniors, focusing on enhancing flexibility, improving balance, and fostering relaxation. Regular practice can lead to improved overall well-being and increased mobility.

10-Minute Daily Flexibility and Balance Routine for Seniors

Note: Use a sturdy chair or wall for support if needed. Perform each exercise slowly and maintain steady breathing.

Toe Touches (2 minutes):

Stand tall, feet hip-width apart, slowly bend forward at the waist, reaching towards your toes. Hold for a few seconds and return to standing.

Benefit: Improves hamstring flexibility and overall balance.

Leg Swings (2 minutes each side):

Stand beside a chair for support, swing one leg forward and backward in a controlled motion. Switch to the other leg.

Benefit: Enhances hip flexibility and improves balance control.

Heel-to-Toe Walk (2 minutes):

Walk in a straight line, placing the heel of one foot directly in front of the toes of the other foot with each step.

Benefit: Enhances balance, coordination, and proprioception.

Standing Quadriceps Stretch (2 minutes each leg):

Stand near a wall for balance, grab one ankle and gently pull towards your buttocks. Switch to the other leg.

Benefit: Stretches the front thigh muscles, improves balance, and flexibility.

Arm Circles (2 minutes):

Stand tall, extend arms to the sides, and make slow circular motions with both arms.

Benefit: Increases shoulder flexibility and improves upper body balance.

Focus on consistent breathing and maintaining proper posture throughout the routine. Individuals should perform these exercises within their comfort level and stop if they experience any discomfort or pain. This routine aims to enhance flexibility, balance, and stability, crucial for preventing falls and maintaining overall mobility.

Recognize the importance of gradual progression and safety during exercises. If individuals have specific health concerns or medical conditions, it's advisable to consult with a healthcare professional before starting any new exercise routine.

30-Minute Daily Flexibility and Balance Routine

Note: Use a sturdy chair or wall for support if needed. Perform each exercise slowly and mindfully, ensuring steady breathing throughout.

Seated Forward Bend (3 minutes):

· Sit on the floor or a chair, extend legs forward, reach for toes, or shins while keeping the spine elongated. Hold the stretch without bouncing.

Benefits: Stretches hamstrings, lower back, and improves spine flexibility.

Sideways Leg Swing (3 minutes each side):

· Stand beside a chair, swing one leg sideways while keeping the body upright and core engaged. Switch to the other leg.

Benefit: Enhances hip mobility, improves balance, and strengthens leg muscles.

Standing Quadriceps Stretch (3 minutes each leg):

· Stand near a wall or chair for support, grab one ankle and gently pull it towards your buttocks. Repeat on the other leg.

Benefit: Stretches the front thigh muscles, enhances balance, and flexibility.

Gentle Yoga Flow (6 minutes):

· Perform a series of gentle yoga poses like Child's Pose, Cat-Cow, and Warrior I. Hold each pose for a few breaths, transitioning slowly between them.

Benefit: Improves overall flexibility, balance, and relaxation.

*The tabletop position is a foundational yoga pose that forms the basis for many other movements and poses. Here's how to get into tabletop position:

Starting Position:

· Start on your hands and knees on a yoga mat or a comfortable surface. Your knees should be directly under your hips, and your hands should be aligned with your shoulders, wrists under shoulders.

· Spread your fingers wide apart and press them firmly into the mat for stability.

· Your spine should be in a neutral position, neither overly arched nor rounded.

Alignment:

· Keep your back straight and engage your core muscles to support your spine. Your gaze should be downward, your neck aligned with your spine.

Balance and Stability:

· Distribute your weight evenly between your hands and knees, ensuring a stable base. Relax your shoulders away from your ears, keeping them down and back.

Breathing and Engagement:

· Breathe naturally and comfortably while holding this position. Engage your abdominal muscles gently to support your lower back and stabilize your core.

The tabletop position is often used as a starting point for various yoga sequences, including Cat-Cow stretches, balancing poses, and core-strengthening exercises. It's a fundamental pose that helps in building stability, awareness of body alignment, and a strong foundation for further yoga practice.

These yoga poses are beneficial for stretching, flexibility, and strengthening different parts of the body. Here's a breakdown of each:

Child's Pose (Balasana):

Starting Position:

· Begin on your hands and knees in a tabletop position, with your wrists aligned under your shoulders and your knees under your hips.

Execution:

· From tabletop, slowly lower your hips back towards your heels.

· Extend your arms in front of you or rest them alongside your body, whichever is more comfortable.

· Lower your forehead to the mat.

· Relax your whole body, allowing your chest to sink towards the floor.

Breathing:

· Breathe deeply into your back, feeling the stretch in your spine, hips, and thighs.

· Hold the pose for 1-3 minutes or longer, maintaining slow, deep breaths.

Cat-Cow Pose (Chakravakasana):

Starting Position:

· Begin in the tabletop position, with your wrists aligned under your shoulders and your knees under your hips.

Execution—Cat Pose:

· As you exhale, round your spine upward towards the ceiling.

· Tuck your chin to your chest and draw your belly button toward your spine.

· Feel the stretch along your back and spine.

Execution—Cow Pose:

· As you inhale, arch your back in the opposite direction.

· Lift your chest and tailbone towards the ceiling, allowing your belly to sink towards the floor.

· Lift your head and gaze forward or slightly upward.

Flow:

· Alternate between Cat and Cow poses, syncing the movement with your breath.

· Move through this sequence for 5-10 breath cycles or as long as comfortable.

Warrior I Pose (Virabhadrasana I):

Starting Position:

· Begin in a standing position at the front of your mat.

· Step one foot back, keeping the front foot facing forward and the back foot at about a 45-degree angle.

· Square your hips toward the front of the mat.

Execution:

· Bend your front knee to a 90-degree angle, ensuring it aligns over your ankle (don't let your knee go past your toes).

· Keep the back leg straight, pressing the outer edge of the back foot into the mat.

· Lift your arms overhead, palms facing each other or touching.

Alignment:

· Lengthen your spine, engaging your core muscles.

· Relax your shoulders away from your ears.

· Gaze forward or slightly upward.

Hold and Breathing:

· Hold the pose for 30 seconds to 1 minute, maintaining steady breathing.

· Repeat on the other side by switching the position of your feet.

Remember, these poses should be done mindfully and within your comfort zone. Gradually deepen into each pose as your body allows, and always listen to your body's signals. It's beneficial to practice under the guidance of a qualified yoga instructor, especially if you're new to yoga or have any physical limitations.

Heel-to-Toe Walking (5 minutes):

· Walk in a straight line, placing the heel of one foot directly in front of the toes of the other foot with each step. Use a chair or wall for support if needed.

Benefit: Enhances balance, coordination, and proprioception.

Hip Flexor Stretch (3 minutes each side):

· Kneel on one knee, lunge forward while keeping the other knee bent at 90 degrees. Lean into the stretch without arching the back. Repeat on the other side.

Benefit: Stretches the hip flexors, improves hip mobility, and balance.

Standing Arm Swings (4 minutes):

· Stand tall, gently swing both arms forward and backward in a controlled manner.

Benefit: Increases shoulder flexibility, improves upper body balance.

Remember to maintain proper form, listen to your body, and avoid overexertion. This routine aims to enhance overall flexibility, improve balance, and contribute to better mobility and stability. Always perform exercises within your comfort level and consult with a healthcare professional before starting any new exercise routine, especially if you have specific health concerns or medical conditions.

8

Chapter 8

Increasing Cardiovascular Endurance

This chapter highlights exercises beneficial for cardiovascular health, educating readers on their importance and how to effectively incorporate them into daily routines. Explains the significance of cardiovascular endurance and its benefits, focusing on exercises promoting heart health. This structured approach ensures comprehensive coverage of various exercises to enhance cardiovascular endurance, emphasizing their importance and practical utilization for senior adults.

Low-Impact Aerobic Exercises

Brisk Walking:

Instructions: Walk briskly for 10-15 minutes, swinging arms naturally and maintaining an upright posture.

Benefit:: Improves cardiovascular health, strengthens bones, and boosts mood.

Swimming Laps:

Instructions: Swim laps at a comfortable pace for 10 minutes, incorporating different strokes like freestyle or breaststroke.

Benefit: Offers a full-body workout, enhances heart health, and minimizes stress on joints.

Cycling (Stationary or Outdoor):

Instructions: Cycle steadily for 10-15 minutes, adjusting resistance as needed for comfort.

Benefit:: Improves cardiovascular fitness, leg strength, and joint mobility.

Water Aerobics:

Instructions: Engage in water aerobics, including leg lifts, arm circles, and water jogging, for 10-15 minutes.

Benefit: Gentle on joints, enhances flexibility, and improves heart health.

Dancing:

Instructions: Dance to your favorite music for 10 minutes, incorporating steps like side steps, grapevines, or simple choreography.

Benefit: Enhances cardiovascular endurance, balance, and coordination.

Elliptical Trainer:

Instructions: Use an elliptical machine for 10-15 minutes, adjusting resistance and speed for comfort.

Benefit: Low-impact on joints, provides a full-body workout, and improves heart rate.

Tai Chi:

Instructions: Practice Tai Chi movements slowly and deliberately for

10 minutes, focusing on fluidity and breathing.

Benefit: Enhances cardiovascular fitness, flexibility, and mental relaxation.

Rowing (Machine or Water):

Instructions: Row steadily for 10 minutes, using proper form by pushing and pulling the handles.

Benefit: Engages upper and lower body muscles, improves heart health, and is low-impact.

These low-impact aerobic exercises offer a range of options to improve cardiovascular health while being gentle on the joints, ensuring a safer and more enjoyable workout routine for seniors.

Seated Jumping Jack Variations

Seated Jumping Jacks:

Instructions: Sit upright in a chair, extend arms to the sides, and simultaneously raise legs outward while clapping hands overhead.

Benefit: Boosts heart rate, improves circulation, and engages arm and leg muscles.

Alternating Arm Raises:

Instructions: Sit tall, raise one arm overhead while lifting the opposite leg out to the side, alternating sides.

Benefit: Enhances cardiovascular endurance and promotes balance and coordination.

Cross-Body Reach:

Instructions: Sitting straight, extend one arm across the body to touch the opposite knee while lifting the same-side leg slightly.

Benefit: Increases heart rate, improves core strength, and engages oblique muscles.

Seated Leg Raises:

Instructions: Sit on the edge of a chair, lift both legs together straight out in front, and lower them back down.

Benefit: Stimulates blood flow, strengthens abdominal muscles, and improves leg endurance.

Toe Taps:

Instructions: Sit tall, tap one foot on the floor in front, then quickly switch to tap the other foot, alternating rapidly.

Benefit: Elevates heart rate, enhances lower body circulation, and encourages foot coordination.

Seated High Knees:

Instructions: Sit upright, bring one knee toward the chest, then alternate quickly between legs, lifting knees as high as comfortable.

Benefit: Increases heart rate, strengthens hip flexors, and improves lower abdominal strength.

Seated Bicycle Kicks:

Instructions: Sit comfortably, lean back slightly, and mimic a cycling motion by pedaling legs alternately.

Benefit: Boosts heart rate, engages core muscles, and promotes lower body flexibility.

Arm Circles with Leg Extension:

Instructions: Extend legs forward while simultaneously making large circles with both arms in a controlled manner.

Benefit: Elevates heart rate, enhances arm and shoulder mobility, and improves leg muscle endurance.

These seated jumping jack variations offer a diverse range of exercises to increase heart rate and improve cardiovascular endurance while being seated, ensuring a safer and effective workout for seniors.

Walking and Marching Variations

Brisk Walking in Place:

Instructions: Stand upright, lift knees higher than normal, and pump arms while briskly walking in place.

Benefit: *Increases heart rate, enhances blood circulation, and improves lower body strength.*

Side Steps:

Instructions: Take sideways steps to the right for a few paces, then return to the starting position and repeat on the left side.

Benefit: *Engages hip muscles, improves lateral movement, and elevates heart rate.*

High Knee Marching:

Instructions: Lift knees higher than usual while marching in place, swinging arms in coordination with the leg movement.

Benefit: *Boosts heart rate, strengthens core muscles, and improves balance and coordination.*

Forward and Backward Walking:

Instructions: Walk forward for a few paces, then switch to walking backward, taking small steps with caution.

Benefit: *Enhances agility, challenges coordination, and engages different leg muscles.*

Heel-to-Toe Walk:

Instructions: Walk by placing the heel of one foot directly in front of the toes of the other foot, taking slow and deliberate steps.

Benefit: *Enhances balance, strengthens leg muscles, and improves stability* *while walking.*

Step Touches:

Instructions: Step to the side with one foot, then bring the other foot to meet it, alternating sides in a rhythmic manner.

Benefit: *Elevates heart rate, enhances coordination, and engages leg muscles.*

Knee Lift and Kickbacks:

Instructions: Lift one knee towards the chest, then extend the leg backward while leaning slightly forward.

Benefit: *Engages core muscles, improves balance, and strengthens the quadriceps and hamstrings.*

Crossover Steps:

Instructions: Step one foot over the other while crossing in front or behind the opposite leg, alternating sides.

Benefit: *Engages hip muscles, challenges coordination, and improves lateral movement.*

These walking and marching variations provide diverse options to increase heart rate, improve circulation, and strengthen various muscle groups, ensuring a comprehensive cardiovascular workout for seniors.

Swimming Techniques for Cardiovascular Health

Given the complexity of describing swimming exercises in detail, I'll offer a general overview of swimming techniques that can enhance cardiovascular health:

Freestyle Stroke:

Instructions: Swim continuously, using alternating arm strokes and flutter kicks while keeping your body streamlined.

Benefit: *Enhances overall cardiovascular endurance, strengthens upper and lower body muscles, and improves breathing capacity.*

Breaststroke:

Instructions: Glide through the water using simultaneous arm movements (circular) and frog-like kicks.

Benefit: Improves heart health, engages core muscles, and is gentle on joints due to its fluid motion.

Backstroke:

Instructions: Float on your back and perform alternating arm movements while flutter kicking.

Benefit: Enhances posture, engages back and shoulder muscles, and provides a great cardiovascular workout.

Butterfly Stroke:

Instructions: Use simultaneous arm movements (both arms come out of the water together) and dolphin kicks.

Benefit: Challenges cardiovascular endurance, strengthens chest and shoulder muscles, and improves coordination.

Treading Water:

Instructions: Maintain a vertical position in the water by moving your arms and legs to stay afloat.

Benefit: Elevates heart rate, improves endurance, and works various muscle groups.

Interval Training:

Instructions: Alternate between fast and slow laps or strokes, incorporating bursts of higher intensity swimming.

Benefit: Enhances cardiovascular fitness, boosts metabolism, and increases overall stamina.

Swimming offers a comprehensive cardiovascular workout by engaging multiple muscle groups simultaneously while being gentle on the joints. It's *an excellent way to improve heart health and overall fitness for seniors.*

Stationary Bike Exercises

Warm-Up Ride:

Instructions: Start pedaling at a low resistance and moderate pace for 5 minutes.

Benefit: Prepares the body for more intense exercise, increases blood flow, and gently elevates heart rate.

Interval Training:

Instructions: Alternate between periods of moderate cycling and short bursts of faster pedaling for 30 seconds to 1 minute each.

Benefit: Boosts cardiovascular fitness, enhances metabolism, and improves endurance.

Hill Climbing Simulation:

Instructions: Increase resistance gradually to simulate climbing a hill; maintain a steady pace.

Benefit: Builds leg strength, increases heart rate, and challenges cardiovascular endurance.

Reverse Pedaling:

Instructions: Pedal backward at a moderate pace for 5-10 minutes.

Benefit: Engages different leg muscles, particularly the hamstrings, and improves balance and coordination.

Steady-State Ride:

Instructions: Maintain a consistent pace and resistance level for 20-30 minutes.

Benefit: Improves cardiovascular endurance, enhances lung capacity, and burns calories steadily.

Sprint Intervals:

Instructions: Alternate between high-intensity sprints (pedaling as fast as comfortable) and recovery periods at a slower pace.

Benefit: Increases heart rate, strengthens leg muscles, and enhances overall cardiovascular fitness.

Seated Climb:

Instructions: Increase resistance and simulate a climb by pedaling in a seated position for 5-10 minutes.

Benefit: Strengthens quadriceps and glutes, improves endurance, and elevates heart rate.

Cool-Down Ride:

Instructions: Lower resistance and pedal at a relaxed pace for 5-10 minutes.

Benefit: Gradually lowers heart rate, helps prevent dizziness, and aids in muscle recovery.

Stationary biking offers a low-impact, effective cardiovascular workout for seniors, allowing for various intensities and styles to suit individual fitness levels.

10-Minute Daily Routine
for Cardiovascular Health

Warm-Up (2 minutes): Begin pedaling at a low resistance and moderate pace for 2 minutes.

Safety Measures: Ensure proper bike setup, sit comfortably, and maintain good posture. Start with low resistance to prevent strain.

Benefit: Prepares the body for exercise, increases blood flow, and gradually raises heart rate.

Interval Training (2 minutes): Alternate between 30 seconds of faster pedaling (increased resistance if comfortable) and 1 minute of moderate-paced cycling.

Safety Measures: Listen to your body; maintain a pace that feels challenging but sustainable. Avoid sudden increases in intensity if you're not used to it.

Benefit: Boosts heart rate, improves cardiovascular endurance, and increases calorie burn.

Steady-State Ride (3 minutes): Maintain a consistent pace and resistance level for 3 minutes.

Safety Measures: Check posture and maintain a smooth pedal stroke to prevent unnecessary strain on joints.

Benefit: Improves endurance, strengthens leg muscles, and further elevates heart rate.

Seated Climb (2 minutes): Increase resistance slightly and pedal in a seated position as if climbing a hill.

Safety Measures: Maintain a controlled and steady pace, avoid jerky movements, and breathe steadily.

Benefit: Strengthens lower body muscles, particularly quadriceps and glutes, and challenges cardiovascular endurance.

Cool-Down (1 minute): Reduce resistance and pedal at a relaxed pace for 1 minute.

Safety Measures: Gradually reduce the intensity to avoid sudden drops in heart rate, preventing dizziness.

Benefit: Aids in muscle recovery, lowers heart rate gradually, and helps prevent stiffness.

This 10-minute routine offers a balanced cardiovascular workout on a stationary bike, focusing on varied intensities to challenge the heart and leg muscles while considering safety for senior adults.

30-Minute Daily Routine for Cardiovascular Health

Warm-Up (5 minutes): Start with a gentle 5-minute ride at a low resistance to warm up muscles and increase blood flow.

Safety Measures: Check bike settings, maintain proper posture, and start with a comfortable resistance level to prevent strain.

Benefit: Prepares the body for exercise, increases heart rate gradually, and reduces the risk of injury.

Interval Training (5 minutes): Alternate between 1 minute of high-intensity pedaling (moderate resistance) and 2 minutes of moderate-paced cycling.

Safety Measures: Adjust intensity gradually, ensuring it feels challenging but manageable. Avoid overexertion.

Benefit: Boosts cardiovascular endurance, elevates heart rate, and burns calories effectively.

Hill Simulation (5 minutes): Gradually increase resistance to simulate a hill climb. Pedal steadily in a seated position.

Safety Measures: Maintain a controlled and steady pace; avoid sudden increases in resistance to prevent strain.

Benefit: Strengthens leg muscles, particularly quadriceps and glutes, and challenges cardiovascular endurance.

Reverse Pedaling (5 minutes): Pedal backward at a moderate pace for 5 minutes to engage different leg muscles.

Safety Measures: Ensure a comfortable pace and a smooth pedal stroke. Be cautious while changing directions.

Benefit: Works different muscle groups, particularly hamstrings, and enhances balance and coordination.

Sprint Intervals (5 minutes): Alternate between 30 seconds of intense pedaling and 1 minute of relaxed cycling.

Safety Measures: Listen to your body; maintain a challenging but sustainable pace. Avoid abrupt changes in speed.

Benefit: Increases heart rate, improves cardiovascular fitness, and boosts metabolism.

Cool-Down (5 minutes): Reduce resistance gradually and pedal at a slow, relaxed pace for the last 5 minutes.

Safety Measures: Gradually reduce intensity to prevent sudden drops in heart rate, preventing dizziness.

Benefit: Aids in muscle recovery, lowers heart rate gradually, and prevents stiffness.

This 30-minute routine offers a comprehensive cardiovascular workout on a stationary bike, focusing on varied intensities while ensuring safety for senior adults.

9

Chapter 9

Progress and Improvements

This chapter aims to empower readers with strategies to monitor their progress, customize their workouts, and seek professional advice, ensuring safe and effective advancements in their fitness journey.

Gradual Intensity Increases

Gradually increasing workout intensity is crucial for overall health improvement. Here are guidelines to recognize when and how to progress within your workout routine:

• **Monitoring Physical Responses:** Pay attention to how your body responds during and after workouts. If you're consistently feeling less fatigued or completing exercises with ease, it might be time to step up the intensity.

• **Assessing Performance:** Keep track of your workout performance. If you find that you're completing exercises more comfortably or have better endurance, it could indicate that you're ready for a progression.

• **Monitoring Heart Rate:** Tracking heart rate during workouts can guide intensity adjustments. If your heart rate becomes consistently lower during a similar exercise, consider increasing intensity to keep it within a target zone for cardiovascular benefit.

• **Exercise Duration and Frequency:** Gradually increase either the duration or frequency of your workouts. For example, extend a workout session by a few minutes or add an extra session per week.

• **Progressive Overload Principle:** Apply the concept of progressive overload by slightly increasing resistance, repetitions, or sets for strength exercises, or elevating speed or duration for cardio workouts.

• **Recovery and Adaptation:** Ensure adequate recovery time between workouts to allow the body to adapt. If you recover well and feel ready for more, it might be time to add intensity.

• **Consulting a Professional:** Seeking advice from a fitness professional can provide structured plans for progression, ensuring safe and effective intensity increases.

Remember, the key is gradual progression. Small increments in intensity will challenge your body without causing strain or injury. Always listen to your body and progress at a pace that feels comfortable yet challenging. This subsection provides practical guidelines for recognizing signs indicating when and how to increase workout intensity, emphasizing the importance of gradual progress for overall health benefits.

Individual Exercise Plans

Designing a personalized exercise plan involves several considerations to optimize overall health and fitness. Here are guidelines to help determine exercises and their scheduling:

• Assess Personal Goals: Define clear fitness objectives, whether it's weight management, improving endurance, building strength, or enhancing flexibility.

• Understanding Personal Limitations: Consider any physical limitations or health concerns. Modify exercises to accommodate these limitations or seek professional guidance for suitable alternatives.

• Balanced Workout Routine: Incorporate a mix of cardiovascular, strength training, flexibility, and balance exercises. For instance:

• Cardiovascular: Engage in aerobic exercises like walking, swimming, or cycling.

• Strength Training: Include resistance exercises using body weight, resistance bands, or weights.

• Flexibility and Balance: Incorporate stretching, yoga, or Tai Chi-inspired movements.

• Progressive Approach: Gradually increase the difficulty or intensity of exercises over time to challenge the body and prevent plateaus.

• Routine Structure: Devise a weekly schedule. For example:

• Cardio Days: Allocate specific days for cardiovascular exercises to improve endurance (e.g., Monday, Wednesday, Friday).

• Strength Training Days: Dedicate separate days for strength exercises to build muscle (e.g., Tuesday, Thursday, Saturday).

• Rest and Recovery: Allow at least one or two days for complete rest or gentle activities to promote recovery.

• Listening to the Body: Pay attention to how the body responds to different exercises and adjust the plan accordingly. If feeling fatigued or sore, allow for additional rest or modify the routine.

• Regular Review: Periodically reassess fitness goals and make necessary adjustments to the exercise plan to ensure continued progress.

• Professional Input: Consult a fitness trainer or healthcare professional to tailor an exercise plan according to individual needs and health status.

Remember, an effective exercise plan is adaptable, balanced, and aligned with personal goals and capabilities.

This section offers guidance on crafting individual exercise plans that suit individual health goals, schedules, and fitness levels, ensuring a comprehensive and tailored approach to overall health improvement.

Professional Guidance

Seeking professional assistance is invaluable for creating a safe and effective exercise routine. Here are guidelines for obtaining professional guidance:

• **Assessment by a Fitness Professional:** Schedule an assessment with a certified fitness trainer or exercise physiologist. They can evaluate your current fitness level, discuss health goals, and design a suitable exercise plan.

• **Consultation with a Healthcare Provider:** If dealing with specific health concerns or conditions, seek advice from a healthcare professional, such as a physician or physical therapist. They can provide insights into exercises that align with your health status.

• **Utilizing Community Resources:** Explore local community centers, gyms, or senior centers that offer fitness programs tailored for older adults. These facilities often have trained staff to guide exercise routines.

• **Online Resources and Apps:** Utilize reputable fitness apps or online platforms offering exercise routines for seniors. Ensure they are endorsed by fitness professionals or health organizations for reliability.

• **Workshops or Group Classes:** Participate in workshops or group exercise classes specifically designed for seniors. These settings provide social support and professional guidance simultaneously.

• **Trusted Referrals:** Seek recommendations from friends, family, or healthcare providers for reputable fitness professionals or programs specialized in senior fitness.

• **Regular Check-ins:** Maintain periodic check-ins with your fitness professional or healthcare provider to review progress, modify routines, and address any concerns.

Remember, professional guidance ensures exercises are tailored to individual needs, minimizes the risk of injury, and maximizes health benefits. This section emphasizes the importance of seeking professional assistance to design safe and effective exercise plans tailored to individual health needs and goals, promoting a holistic approach to overall health improvement.

10

Conclusion

As we close the chapters on "Top 50+ Exercises for Senior Adults," it's crucial to reflect on the essential elements that define this journey towards improved health and well-being.

Recap of Key Points:

Throughout these pages, we've explored the significance of exercise in the lives of seniors. From understanding the physical benefits that exercise offers to unraveling its profound impact on mental and emotional well-being, the aim has been to equip you with insights that empower and inspire.

Let me encourage you to Stay Active:

Remember, this journey towards better health is ongoing. Embracing an active lifestyle isn't just about physical fitness; it's a commitment to nurturing every aspect of your well-being. Consistency and dedication pave the way for a more vibrant and fulfilling life.

Resources for Further Support:

As you continue on this path, seek out local community centers, senior fitness programs, or online resources tailored to senior adults.

Additionally, consider consulting fitness professionals or healthcare providers for personalized guidance and support in your fitness endeavors.

Your feedback is invaluable! If this book has contributed positively to your fitness journey, sharing your thoughts through an Amazon review can help guide and motivate others on their path to improved senior fitness.

Remember, age isn't a limitation; it's an opportunity to prioritize your health and well-being. Embrace movement, embrace strength, and continue enriching your life through the power of exercise.

Thank you for embarking on this journey with me. Here's to a healthier, happier, and more active you!